SO MUCH TO BE DONE

So Much to Be Done

THE WRITINGS OF BREAST CANCER ACTIVIST BARBARA BRENNER

BARBARA BRENNER

EDITED BY **BARBARA SJOHOLM**
INTRODUCTION BY **RACHEL MORELLO-FROSCH**
AFTERWORD BY **ANNE LAMOTT**

University of Minnesota Press
Minneapolis • London

Writing in Part I was previously published in *The Source*, a newsletter of Breast Cancer Action. Writing in Part II previously appeared in Healthy Barbs at http://barbarabrenner.net/ or on Barbara Brenner's Caring Bridge website at http://www.caringbridge.org/visit/barbarabrenner.

"Gott spricht zu jedem . . . / God speaks to each of us . . ." from Rainer Maria Rilke, *Rilke's Book of Hours: Love Poems to God*, translated by Anita Barrows and Joanna Macy (New York: Riverhead, 1996), 88. Translation copyright 1996 by Anita Barrows and Joanna Macy. Reprinted by permission of the translators and of Riverhead, an imprint of Penguin Publishing Group, a division of Penguin Random House LLC.

"Dance Me to the End of Love," by Leonard Cohen, excerpted from *Stranger Music: Selected Poems and Songs*. Copyright 1993 by Leonard Cohen. Reprinted by permission of McClelland and Stewart, a division of Penguin Random House Canada Limited.

"Mi Shebeirach" music copyright 1989 by The Deborah Lynn Friedman Trust, Dated October 19, 1994; text by Deborah Friedman and Drorah Setel (based on liturgy).

Published by the University of Minnesota Press
111 Third Avenue South, Suite 290
Minneapolis, MN 55401-2520
http://www.upress.umn.edu

ISBN 978-0-8166-9943-8 (hc) | ISBN 978-0-8166-9944-5 (pb)
A Cataloging-in-Publication record is available from the Library of Congress.

Printed in the United States of America on acid-free paper

The University of Minnesota is an equal-opportunity educator and employer.

23 22 21 20 19 18 17 16   10 9 8 7 6 5 4 3 2 1

Contents

A Portrait of Barbara Brenner

Barbara Sjoholm

Most breast cancer activists will have heard of Barbara Brenner, and many will have seen her as a participant in the documentary *Pink Ribbons, Inc.*, which skewered corporate pinkwashing and other hypocrisies in the multimillion-dollar breast cancer industry. There are those who read her columns in Breast Cancer Action's newsletters or reached out to her personally for advice and help. Many followed her blog, Healthy Barbs, for information and back talk on breast cancer and other health issues or drew comfort and strength from her posts about her struggles with ALS, the disease that eventually took her life in 2013. But others will be encountering Barbara Brenner for the first time in this selection of writings from her editorial columns and blog posts. A self-described "hell-raiser," Barbara Brenner was for fifteen years the executive director of the San Francisco–based organization Breast Cancer Action, which she described with relish as "the bad girls of breast cancer."

In Barbara Brenner's mind a *hell-raiser* was a question-asker, an agent of change, and a dogged and courageous pursuer of truth, all elements of her own personality that she managed to combine with humor and great energy. Readers of this selection of Barbara's columns and blog posts will have the opportunity to experience directly just what made Barbara such a galvanizing and sometimes controversial figure in the world of breast cancer research and health activism. As one of her friends and colleagues, Peggy Orenstein, wrote: "Barbara was the person who most influenced my own thinking and writing

1

about breast cancer. Often, in fact, she was so far ahead of the rest of us in her understanding of the disease and its politics that I privately thought her a tad extreme. Only now is the rest of the world catching up to where she was over a decade ago on critical issues."

Barbara Brenner, who would become such a powerful voice for activist health issues as the director of Breast Cancer Action, was born in Baltimore in 1951. She grew up, one of seven children, in a large rambling house in the northwest corner of the city, the "self-created Jewish ghetto," as she described it. In one of her earliest memories she wanted to go out and play in the snow with her big brother and sister. She was three years old. Her mother said no, and she responded: "'Oh wes I are,' and out I went. I guess no was not an answer I liked even as a little kid."

Baltimore helped shape her views of social justice. "Segregation of blacks was intense. There was, thank goodness, an active civil rights movement; my mother was involved with it. She took me to my first civil rights march when I was about ten. That's where I first saw Martin Luther King Jr." She went to public schools from kindergarten through high school, even though her mother would have preferred that she attend the all-girls' academic high school downtown. "I said no. She slugged me with her shoe. I won the battle and had a black eye to prove it." In high school Barbara first found a lump in her left breast; she had an excisional biopsy, and the lump was found to be benign. With her parents often fighting, Barbara discovered freedom in a driver's license. "My parents would start in, and I would get in the car and drive." Staying in Baltimore for college was not appealing. Based on the catalog from Smith College ("no pictures, just pages and pages of course descriptions"), she applied, was accepted, and received generous financial aid.

At Smith she majored in government, because already she knew she wanted to be a lawyer—and had known since she was six, when her uncle died. He had been a lawyer who had helped create the International Monetary Fund. She also became involved in antiwar activities, participating in teach-ins and organizing events. Her junior year was spent in Geneva, Switzerland, where she became fluent in French, though she never mastered downhill skiing. She had a boyfriend, but the relationship ended during her senior year. "He didn't want me to apply to top-notch law schools because I might take a place more needed by a guy who was going to have to support a family." Instead she fell in love with another woman student at Smith. ("I didn't call myself a lesbian then; the person I loved happened to be a woman.") She then moved to Washington, D.C., to attend Georgetown University's law school, where she learned, "to my horror, that law and justice were not synonymous." After a year she left Georgetown to attend the Woodrow Wilson School of Public and International Affairs at Princeton University. She was so sure law school was behind her that she sold all her textbooks.

At Princeton she met Susie Lampert, a fellow student who would become her life partner. "My immediate impression was, 'She's a dyke.' Susie's immediate impression of me was, 'She comes on like a train.'" Throughout the fall they played endless games of Scrabble, as both recognized that to act on their feelings would mean they were lesbians. "That seemed like a big deal to me at the age of twenty-three," Barbara recalled, but of course it was: "We were two women falling in love at one of the most sexist, homophobic institutions in the country. Between that stark reality and the uncertainty that a same-sex relationship posed for each of us, neither of us was ready to move quickly." Yet "the more I thought about my love for Susie, the more radicalized [I became] in my thinking about the role of women in society and the traditional place reserved for them in primary relationships with men. I began to understand that I was a lesbian and that that had implications for how [I] was perceived and [how I] behaved in the world. I was waking up politically in ways that astonished me. I thought I had been politicized by the Vietnam War. I'm certain that my activities [were] influenced by [my] growth as a radical feminist."

Susie had grown up in Los Angeles, and after she earned a master's degree in public affairs and urban planning, the new couple moved to the West Coast, staying with Susie's parents at first. Barbara, who had left Princeton without a degree, went to work as a law clerk for Jill Jakes, who ran the Southern California ACLU's Women's Rights Project. "Jill was willing to let me do anything I was capable of doing, so I got a lot of experience researching and writing up legal issues, drafting briefs, and talking to prospective clients." Her favorite case was *Weathers v. the Superior Court of Los Angeles County*, which established for the first time under California law that a woman did not automatically take her husband's name when she married.

In 1976, the couple decided to move to San Francisco and, with help from Susie's parents, they bought a house in Noe Valley. Susie was able to find work in her field as a city planner, and Barbara took a job with the Bay Area Feminist Federal Credit Union. Although the job was short-lived, she made important connections with a number of lesbian feminists in the Bay Area. "That's how we got connected to the 1978 statewide fight over the Briggs Initiative. This was a proposal to ban gay and lesbian teachers from the public schools. Anita Bryant, the orange juice queen from Florida, got involved on the other side of that battle. We won that one."

Barbara decided to return to law school, this time at Berkeley Law School (then called Boalt Hall). She quickly became involved with the women's caucus at Boalt, making friends for life. Her first summer job was at the ACLU of Northern California, where she spent much of her time helping prepare a challenge to a California statute that required teenage girls to get permission from their parents in order to have an abortion. "I worked with great lawyers interviewing and gathering declarations from medical experts about the impact of the law on teenagers." She was also strongly influenced by the ACLU's approach to protecting civil liberties.

Her second summer job was with the legal firm of Rosen, Remcho and Henderson. Barbara said she learned one of her most important lessons as an activist and organizer from Sandy Rosen: "Sandy had sent me to the library to research how he might get around a certain court order issued to his client. I did the research and called Sandy to explain what the law did not allow. Sandy said, 'That's fine. You told me what I can't do. Now figure out what I can do.'"

In 1980, Barbara was asked by another member of the legal firm, Thelton Henderson, who had just been nominated as a federal court judge and was awaiting confirmation, if she would be willing to serve as his law clerk after she finished law school: "Yes was the only conceivable answer." With Judge Henderson she found a friend and mentor who gave her and his other clerk lots of responsibility as researchers who would then discuss their recommendations and make a decision. After her year as a clerk, she joined the firm of Remcho, Johansen and Purcell (RJP) and worked on several large cases until 1986, when she joined Donna Hitchens, the founding lawyer of the Lesbian Rights Project, to create the firm Hitchens and Brenner. The practice closed in 1990 after Donna ran for judicial office and was elected. Barbara returned to RJP, first as a special counsel and then as a partner. During this time Barbara grew increasingly active as a board member with the ACLU of Northern California and then as a board member nationally. She credited her experience with the ACLU as giving her a deep understanding of how organizations worked, something that would soon become important in her involvement at Breast Cancer Action.

Barbara loved her work and most likely would have continued to thrive as a progressive lawyer if not for the fact that in the fall of 1993 she discovered a lump in her left breast during a routine self-exam. Her surgeon did a needle biopsy that was inconclusive, then a biopsy. "I had the biopsy in August, just before Susie's forty-third birthday. I remember sitting over a lovely dinner at L'Avenue Restaurant talking about what if this turned out to be cancer. At that point, it was a theoretical discussion." Soon after that dinner, the surgeon confirmed the lump was malignant, and Barbara's life, like that of so many women who hear the same news, changed radically.

From the moment Barbara heard the diagnosis, delivered reluctantly and without much information by a doctor who answered the first question she had on her list ("What kind of cancer is it?") with a patronizing "You don't need to know that," she found ways to act on her own behalf, an attitude she had had from childhood and one that had been strengthened by her legal training and work with progressive lawyers on important rights cases. As she would write again and again over the next decades, activism is "not for the faint of heart." In Barbara's case, activism was a way of life that stood her in good stead for many years as she worked first to understand her own illness, and then the breast cancer experiences of other women, and finally the large and small issues that made it so difficult to grapple with and confront a corporate breast cancer industry that grew up in tandem with one of the major health epidemics of our time.

Barbara came to Breast Cancer Action (BCA, now BCAction) when the organization was four years old and had one half-time paid staff person. In early 1994, while she was still in chemotherapy, Barbara published a letter in the *San Francisco Chronicle* objecting to a lead editorial that argued against devoting more money to breast cancer research when the facts showed more women die of heart disease and lung cancer than of breast cancer. The day her letter ran she received a call from Nancy Evans, then president of the board of Breast Cancer Action, who asked to meet, saying the organization needed people like her. Barbara hesitated to commit at first, because of her health, but she began writing occasionally for the *BCA Newsletter*. Within a year of being invited to join the board of the organization, she became its president and then the first full-time executive director and began a task she relished, becoming the person who would "whip the organization into shape."

In the beginning Barbara (who had taken to wearing a Stetson hat to cover her short, post-chemo hair, along with her usual clothes, a button-down shirt, blue jeans, and Timberland boots) had to cope with perceptions about being the only out lesbian on the board. Some of the board feared that "if BCA became too identified with lesbians, the organization would become marginalized. But BCA was founded and stayed on the margins of the breast cancer movement. It was a strategy to push the movement more toward where BCA wanted it to go. Lesbians were perfect for that strategy."

Barbara's personality was a good match for the cutting-edge organization, and over the years she would become its public face, a whip-smart, incisive speaker with strong organizational skills and a far-reaching grasp of strategy. She was brilliant, dogged, respected, and, in certain quarters, feared. She would stand up to anyone but usually with an infectious smile and a wisecrack. Her humor perhaps was one of her greatest weapons in puncturing the falsehoods and half-truths that the breast cancer industry fostered.

Barbara Brenner was BCA's executive director for fifteen years, attending conferences, speaking on the radio, and continuing to research and write on the subject of cancer treatments, corporate profits, and health activism. From the beginning she figured out that a media presence would be key to the small organization's success and funding. She always took calls from the press, and soon she saw that attending scientific meetings on the subject of cancer was immensely important, to understand what was being said about research and to ask questions, to "sit near a floor mike and be first in line with a question for the presenter if I had one. I always introduced myself by my name, and BCA's."

She considered her core mission to work against corporate domination of breast cancer and oversimplified messages. This would eventually include a critique of the language of how mammograms save lives and of how cancer drugs are marketed and sold, and would eventually encompass large campaigns critical of Walk for the Cure and other strategies of corporate branding by large companies such as Avon, Estée Lauder, and Ford Motors. As Rachel Morello-Frosch explores in her introduction to this book, it was a long and challenging road to build a movement based on information and activism, all the more to do that with the humor and feistiness for which BCA became known. Campaigns such as Think Before You Pink® brought the issues before the public and inspired many of those living with breast cancer and their supporters to question the messages they heard.

Barbara's initial treatment (a lumpectomy, radiation, and chemotherapy) after her diagnosis in 1993 took eleven months, during which time she left the law practice, first on disability leave and then permanently during the first half of 1995. She took the full-time job at Breast Cancer Action in September 1995. In 1996, she suffered a recurrence of breast cancer and had a mastectomy that fall.

Barbara remained cancer-free after this second occurrence, but with a greater understanding of life's fragility and the importance of making the most of one's time and enjoying life. She practiced the piano every morning before work and left the office at 5 p.m. whenever possible to have time with friends or attend a symphony performance or a play. She and Susie took three-week vacations, often hiking and spending time in nature. Barbara's commitment to her partner, which had begun when they were in their early twenties, became a sustaining part of her life, as did their personal and professional friendships in San Francisco and around the country. Feisty as Barbara was, she recognized early on that relationships were always important to her in her work and reflected, "I'm pretty good at not burning bridges." More than that, she saw community as a value in itself. Being there for friends, some of whom lived with breast cancer, was an integral part of the couple's life. Barbara, who had experienced an outpouring of love and support when she first had breast cancer, was able to reciprocate a hundredfold. She said, "I know that the connections I have made with people over many years of living a public life are the most valuable resource I have other than Susie's love and commitment."

She would have need of her different communities when, in

2010, on the verge of retiring from Breast Cancer Action as she turned sixty, she began to have trouble talking. "Usually in the evening, when I was tired, my words would be slurred. Some people thought I had had too much to drink, but all I had had was water." She saw her doctor and he diagnosed fatigue, but late that fall, after numerous tests, the verdict was clear: she had amyotrophic lateral sclerosis, ALS, a progressive neurodegenerative disease that affects nerve cells in the brain and the spinal cord, causing the muscles to weaken and waste away. Later Barbara would write:

> I had learned when I had breast cancer in 1993 that the line between health and illness is razor thin. During our lives, we cross back and forth often, often not thinking about it—colds, the flu, chicken pox. Even with serious health issues like cancer or heart disease, for example, we sometimes get to cross back to the health side. And then, a day comes when we cross only in one direction.

In October 2010, Breast Cancer Action hosted a large celebration in honor of its twentieth anniversary. Barbara had not yet told the board she had ALS, but her diagnosis meant a more rapid departure from the organization than they had all anticipated. For the next year, she continued to write about breast cancer in a new blog, Healthy Barbs, even as her medical struggles with ALS would increasingly take center stage. She also wrote, often more personally, in the social media blog Caring Bridge. Being Barbara, she didn't take the received wisdom about ALS for granted: "While breast cancer was my introduction to the world of illness, I've discovered since I now have ALS that issues from one illness often have implications for other illnesses, both personally and politically." As she explored what could help her quality of life, from a feeding tube to speech technology, she shared all those experiences online and infused her blog posts with moxie, humor, anger, and compassion. She accepted her situation but not with resignation:

> I think who we are doesn't change because we become ill. I
> have always been a sort of cranky or cynical optimist, and I
> bring that to living with ALS. I know a lot of people who just

give up, moan about what they are losing. I certainly am aware of what I'm losing, but that drives my desire to keep doing whatever I can, as long as I can. I'm amazed at how many people with ALS don't know about or use this speech technology, who want to avoid a feeding tube because it feels too invasive so they risk pneumonia or choking when they try to eat. It's just not my way. I'm not a health activist for nothing.

For herself and Susie and their friends, Barbara kept up a Can Do/Can't Do List, a practical, gratitude-infused inventory of what was possible and was becoming less possible. After more than a year of living with ALS she could write in her Can Do List that she could play the piano, hear songs in her head, sleep with her sweetie, think, help people with breast cancer issues, be an ALS activist, and consider the wonder of the world. What she could not do was sing, talk, eat, or socialize easily. But Barbara found ways to keep communicating through speech technology, writing on her iPad, and typing words that were translated into sound by the iPad apps NeoKate and Speak it! In addition to her blogs, she made notes for a book that would tell her own story and that of the breast cancer activist movement. Although Barbara's own voice was now silent, she had not been silenced, and she continued her activism in whatever ways were available to her.

In May 2012, a documentary by the Canadian director Léa Pool, *Pink Ribbons, Inc.,* based in part on Samantha King's book by the same name, was released by the National Film Board of Canada. The film offered a critique of marketing the color pink to create an impression of corporate caring and to increase profits. At the same time the film explored the language of "the war on breast cancer" and the notion of "fighting for a cure." In reality, research on breast cancer was confusing, opaque, and often repetitious. It was also unclear where the vast amounts of money raised by races, walks, and pink-ribboned merchandise was going, since accountability was limited. Barbara Brenner, along with Samantha King, Barbara Ehrenreich, and Dr. Susan Love, was one of the main voices of the documentary—and one of the most straightforward and spirited. She was able to travel to Northampton, Massachusetts, to introduce a screening of the film at Smith College. She began by asking the audience to raise their hands if they or anyone they knew had breast cancer and then went on:

People say to me that the pink ribbon—on lapels, on products as varied as toilet paper and handguns—helps raise awareness of breast cancer. My argument is that, thanks in part to the pink ribbon, everyone is now aware of breast cancer, unless they are living under a rock. Isn't it time to move beyond awareness to activism to change the course of the epidemic?

If you think doing a walk for breast cancer, or a run, or a mountain climb is the way to end the breast cancer epidemic, the film you are about to see will, I hope, convince you otherwise.

And if buying a product with a pink ribbon on it would help end the epidemic, it should be over by now, given all the breast cancer shopping that people do. After all, if shopping could cure breast cancer, it would be cured by now.

The screening of the film coincided with Smith College's Rally Day, where Barbara, along with four other alumnae, was awarded a Smith College Medal for her work in breast cancer activism. In addition to the medal bestowed by Smith, Barbara received, during the last six months of her life, the Lola Hanzel Courageous Advocacy Award from the American Civil Liberties Union of Northern California (ACLU–NC) at its annual Bill of Rights Day Celebration in December 2013. In her acceptance speech, Barbara spoke about how meaningful volunteering had been to her: "Sooner or later, all issues of social justice are connected. And we as individuals can advance the arc of history towards justice by volunteering. The world changes because we work for change."

In both cases Barbara was able to deliver speeches via Speak it!, giving eloquent voice to the continuing importance of activism in her life. For Barbara, these were occasions to acknowledge the efforts others had made, what she had learned from mentors and colleagues, and how she had tried to put her education and volunteering to a purpose larger than herself.

Barbara identified as Jewish, and she and Susie had always observed the holidays. During the last ten years of her life she began to develop her spirituality more consciously, joining a synagogue with Susie. Community was crucial to Barbara, and Jewish community, with its emphasis on social activism, had been important to her throughout her involvement in many issues over her lifetime. After ALS took hold, she wrote increasingly about Judaism and her faith in her blog posts, particularly on the Caring Bridge site:

> I've taken a Hebrew name because that was important to me, and it's also a Jewish tradition to change one's name to try to fool the angel of death. And I have started studying Torah, which is a fascinating study for an intellectual person like me. We now do Shabbat on Friday nights, and I listen to CDs of people singing Jewish prayers. It feeds a part of my soul. Every morning when I wake up I say to myself the prayer that thanks God for returning my soul to me.

Barbara's faith was both a solace and an interrogation that continued until her death in May 2013. Rabbi Margaret Holub recalled that

> we said a prayer that is customary to say before death. It speaks of the soul finding its eternal rest in the Garden of Eden, under the wing of God. The next day, the day she died, I asked Barbara if there was anything else she wanted to ask or tell me. She typed me a note: what do you mean by the word "soul"?
>
> There is probably a complicated theological answer to give, but what I said in that moment, which I didn't know I knew, which I learned from Barbara, is that our souls, whatever they are, breathed into us at some unknown moment before we are born, are uniquely and distinctively ourselves. Our souls make us who we are. They animate our particular and unique being for whatever time we are given to be here in this world.

Until the end, Barbara Brenner was a question-asker. One of her legacies to us, expressed in the vitality and courage of her writings, is to learn to question and to keep demanding answers, no matter how often we are told it doesn't matter or not to bother. But while Barbara Brenner reveled in saying no when necessary, she was also pragmatic, forward-thinking, and willing to work with people to change their minds. She was not focused only on the can't-do but, life affirmingly, on the can-do. Her engaged and loving activism, which demonstrates what can be done, what can always be done, is her greatest teaching.

Acknowledgments

For bringing me into contact with Susie Lampert and this book project, I thank Phyllis Hatfield, a mutual friend of Susie and Barbara and me. Susie Lampert deserves most of the credit for this book, from initially gathering the material to providing excellent advice and connections. I thank her for trusting me with Barbara's words and for her steadfastness and encouragement. Karuna Jaggar, the current executive director of Breast Cancer Action, gave her whole-hearted backing to the project, and Angela Wall, then BCAction's communications director, put together a collection of the original newsletter columns. Thanks go to Anne Lamott and Rachel Morello-Frosch for their contributions to the book, and to Samantha King for her support. The University of Minnesota Press could not have been a better home for this collection, and many thanks to Danielle Kasprzak, Anne Carter, Laura Westlund, Louisa Castner, Rachel Moeller, Emily Hamilton, Heather Skinner, and all the other fine staff at the Press. Jane Zones encouraged Barbara Brenner to write this book. Caitlin Carmody of BCAction, Elaine Elinson, Simon Frankel, and Roberta Lampert also offered advice and encouragement.

Many quotations from Barbara Brenner in this essay are taken from an unfinished autobiographical manuscript found on her iPad after her death. At the beginning of her manuscript she listed several possible titles for the book, including "Not for the Faint of Heart" and "My Life as a Hell-Raiser." Some information, including dates, has been supplemented by Susie Lampert. Other material is taken from an oral history Barbara did for Smith College (Barbara Brenner interview by Zaylia Pluss, transcript of video recording, April 20, 24, 27, 29, and May 4, 2012, Sophia Smith Collection, Smith College, Northampton, Massachusetts), and the eulogy delivered by Rabbi Margaret Holub at Barbara's funeral.

Barbara Brenner, Breast Cancer Action, and the Birth of a Politicized Breast Cancer Movement

Rachel Morello-Frosch

I first met Barbara Brenner in the late 1980s, when, fresh out of college, I began working for Equal Rights Advocates, a women's rights
law firm in San Francisco. The organization was located in a building filled with other civil rights groups, including the American Civil
Liberties Union of Northern California, where Barbara served as a
board member and prolific fund-raiser. I was a young activist starting
a challenging new job with ERA's Women of Color Project, and many
of the seasoned advocates in that building, including Barbara, became
political mentors who helped me navigate the legal and policy worlds
of civil rights advocacy in the San Francisco Bay Area and nationally.
Three years later, I left my dream job to attend graduate school at UC–
Berkeley, but Barbara, along with her life partner, Susie Lampert, and
I stayed in touch despite our busy lives on opposite sides of the Bay.

In the late summer of 1993, when I was twenty-eight years old and
about to start a doctoral program in environmental health sciences,
I was diagnosed with breast cancer. Within a week of my diagnosis,
Barbara herself found out that she too had the disease. She was forty-
one at the time. During that fateful week, my political mentor became
my "bosomless buddy" as we joined the dreaded sisterhood of breast
cancer and embarked on treatment regimens commonly described as

"slash, burn, and poison." During that year, we shared a lot about grueling breast cancer treatments and their side effects (hair days versus no hair days), feeling underwhelmed about breast cancer support groups and breast cancer organizations that promoted "breast cancer awareness," and coming to terms with the reality that our time on this planet is short and that we had better get on with "living lives that matter," as Barbara liked to say.

Shortly thereafter, in 1994, Barbara got involved with Breast Cancer Action as a board member. By the fall of 1995 she had become the organization's first full-time executive director. BCA (now BCAction) was at the time a small nonprofit, founded in 1990 by a group of women living with breast cancer in the San Francisco Bay Area. Frustrated by the lack of information about the causes and treatment of their disease, these women created an activist group that demanded answers and accountability as well as dispensed information and support to women with breast cancer. BCA's mission was large and its paid staff was small, so it was fortuitous that Barbara, with her legal background and experience as a civil rights advocate and fundraiser, came along. Similarly, it was Barbara's good fortune that BCA enabled her to extend her many organizational skills and develop as a breast cancer activist. Her razor-sharp analysis, capacity to build partnerships with allies and supporters, wicked sense of humor, and uncompromising approach to organizing infused in me and many others a sense of urgency and optimism that made us roll up our sleeves and get to work to end the breast cancer epidemic. Under Barbara's leadership, BCA would grow from a feisty band of activists to a formidable organization with national clout and thousands of members.

Breast Cancer Action's Radical Brand of Cancer Politics

BCA has roots in the feminist and women's health movements of the 1960s and 1970s. These movements fundamentally challenged institutional practices in health care access and delivery, including traditional notions of compliant female patients in relationship to their physicians and other (mostly male) medical "experts." Organizations such as the National Women's Health Network and Our Bodies Ourselves empowered women to become their own health experts and advocates through the dissemination of accessible information and the provision of services that placed women at the center of medical and scientific conversations about their health and well-being. The women's health movement also politically engaged women to address their systemic exclusion from medical education and health care policymaking. Influenced by this movement history, BCA (not surprisingly) quickly distinguished itself as an organization that views breast cancer as public health and social justice issues and seeks to end the breast cancer epidemic through organizing, outreach, and collective action. BCA's advocacy has focused on a critical analysis of environmental policy and scientific research on the causes of and treatment for breast cancer. The organization has also worked to increase health care access for communities disparately impacted by the disease, and to unveil profiteering and conflicts of interest in corporate underwriting of Breast Cancer Awareness Month, multibillion-dollar Shop for the Cure campaigns, and the pink ribbon industry. As executive director, Barbara refined BCA's approach to organizing and action, in order to transform public perception of breast cancer from an individual disease, to be dealt with privately, to a politicized and collective illness experience requiring systemic social and policy change. As BCA grew, its radical and passionate form of political activism contrasted sharply with the traditional nonconfrontational tactics of the mainstream breast cancer movement; this orientation led some observers to dub the organization the "bad girls of breast cancer"— a characterization that Barbara embraced by putting the slogan on a BCA T-shirt.

BCA's origins, similar to those of other breast cancer organizations, can be traced to cancer support groups that have provided emotional and psychological support to those facing the disease's diverse challenges.[1] While many women gravitated toward these groups seeking solidarity and opportunities to share their personal illness experiences, the founders of BCA realized that they needed to collectively mobilize their *politicized illness experience* in order to leverage resources and push for the institutional changes necessary to support true prevention and extend access to effective health care for all women at risk or facing the disease.[2] BCA's approach represented a fundamental shift in health social movement organizing by highlighting the limits of medical science to address the fundamental causes of a disease that was increasing in incidence and that was driven predominantly by social, economic, and environmental factors. Indeed, during the two decades ending in the early 1990s, breast cancer incidence rates rose by an estimated 24 percent, with an average annual increase of 1.7 percent.[3] BCA's founders, along with leaders of other breast cancer advocacy groups that emerged during the same period across the country, were frustrated by the lack of scientific evidence on breast cancer etiology. Women wanted to expand scientific inquiry on breast cancer causation beyond a perennial focus on individual and behavioral risk factors (such as genetics, reproductive history, diet, exercise, and other so-called lifestyle factors), which had thus far yielded equivocal results, to include potential environmental links; the latter was of particular interest to women who were concerned about high breast cancer rates in their communities in several areas across the United States, including Long Island, New York, Cape Cod, Massachusetts, as well as Marin County, Bayview–Hunters Point, and Richmond in Northern California. Bayview and Richmond are both low-income communities of color that have received less media attention than wealthier communities but that have faced significant environmental health challenges due to pollution legacies related to shipbuilding, oil refining, and the power industry. This attention effectively transformed these neighborhoods into epicenters of environmental justice organizing. Breast Cancer Action consistently highlighted the fact that there were many African American women dying at young ages from breast cancer in these communities and that these areas needed more regulatory and scientific attention, due to their proximity to major pollution sources.

In collaboration with environmental, public health and social justice groups, Barbara cultivated BCA's distinct form of activism, which can be characterized as an "embodied health movement" with four elements.[4] First, BCA activists leverage their illness experience as a powerful counterauthority to dominant theories of disease causation within medical science and seek to overturn corporate control over treatment access. Second, BCA confronts the narratives of mainstream cancer organizations, such as the American Cancer Society, about breast cancer as an individual problem and challenges false notions of disease prevention that overemphasize behavioral change and mammography screening. Third, BCA's activism promotes strategic coalition building with other women's health, breast cancer, environmental health, civil rights, and environmental justice organizations. Fourth, collaborating with scientists and health professionals, BCA works to democratize the scientific enterprise and expand research in more fruitful directions, including increasing funding to examine environmental links, elucidate viable paths to prevention, and enhance treatment access to low-income women and women of color.

In their efforts to reframe the conversation about how to end the breast cancer epidemic, BCA's early activists combined tactics adopted from protestors and advocates from the AIDS, environmental, and women's movements and turned those tactics into their own style of direct confrontation with policymakers, research institutions such as the National Institutes of Health, and the pharmaceutical industry. For example, partnering with AIDS activists from ACT UP Golden Gate in the early 1990s, BCA founding members drove onto the lawns of the pharmaceutical company Genentech to demand patient access to Herceptin, then an experimental drug that was pending approval by the Food and Drug Administration. This in-your-face activism ultimately yielded results when, in 1997, Barbara and BCA worked with Genentech to create a landmark "compassionate use" policy under which women with metastatic breast cancer could enter a lottery to receive Herceptin even if they had not been accepted into clinical trials.

Barbara also advanced BCA's efforts to challenge corporate dominance over breast cancer science in the legal arena: in collaboration with the ACLU, BCA successfully dismantled corporate human gene patents. The company Myriad Genetics held patents for more than fifteen years on two genes, BRCA-1 and BRCA-2, that reveal a woman's risk of hereditary breast and ovarian cancer. BCA had tried unsuccessfully to convince Congress to address this issue when patents on these two human genes were first issued. However, as a plaintiff in this historic Supreme Court case, which was decided in 2013, BCA helped end the corporate stranglehold on human genes, which has facilitated data sharing and enhanced the availability of affordable genetic testing for at-risk patients with strong family histories of breast and ovarian cancer. BCA was the only national breast cancer organization to collaborate on this legal case, in part because Barbara leveraged important linkages between breast cancer and civil liberties advocacy and, as she pointed out, "Sooner or later, all issues of social justice are connected."

Challenging Corporate Accountability in the Breast Cancer Industry

Perhaps one of Barbara's key legacies was how she worked to transform breast cancer advocacy by directly challenging corporate funding of the cancer establishment. In 2002, BCA became the first and only breast cancer organization to launch a media and organizing campaign against corporate cause marketing that targeted Breast Cancer Awareness Month, Shop for the Cure, and other forms of pink ribbon fund-raising. Creatively called Think Before You Pink®, the campaign continues to use humor, savvy media strategies, and corporate shaming to highlight egregious cases of industry "pinkwashing." Highlights of this ongoing campaign include exposing Kentucky Fried Chicken's comarketing of pink buckets of chicken with the Susan G. Komen Foundation, a major breast cancer philanthropic organization, which BCA dubbed "What the Cluck?" The organization also successfully pressured General Mills, the manufacturer of Yoplait yogurt, to "Put a Lid On It" and remove growth hormones from their dairy products. Think Before You Pink® changed public and media conversations about corporate profiteering from breast cancer and has been covered nationally in outlets such as the *New York Times*, the *Colbert Report*, the *Daily Show with Jon Stewart*, and the 2013 documentary *Pink Ribbons, Inc.* The campaign received an award from the Business Ethics Network.

Barbara also worked closely with BCA board members to raise ethical questions about conflicts of interest inherent in the corporate funding of breast cancer advocacy. Biotechnology and pharmaceutical companies have long cultivated relationships through philanthropy with breast cancer organizations interested in promoting research to improve treatment outcomes and prevention. Indeed, while pharmaceutical companies and breast cancer groups both want to encourage the development of more effective treatment regimens, new pharmaceutical products, while generally beneficial for the corporate bottom line, may not necessarily help women. Through her speeches and writings, Barbara pushed breast cancer groups to ask themselves, Can a breast cancer organization that receives corporate funding from pharmaceutical companies objectively evaluate and communicate critical information about scientific discoveries and clinical trials of new drug treatments to women dealing with breast cancer?[5] Ultimately, BCA addressed this ethical challenge by adopting a formal policy that rejects funding from companies or entities that profit from cancer or that may be contributing to cancer by polluting the environment. This groundbreaking policy distinguished BCA within the breast cancer movement and the scientific community as an organization that could not be bought and that was free to say and do things that other groups avoided due to fears of jeopardizing their funding.[6] Barbara leveraged BCA's corporate funding policy to challenge other breast cancer organizations and coalitions, including the Susan G. Komen Foundation, the National Breast Cancer Coalition, and the National Alliance of Breast Cancer Organizations, to disclose their own conflicts of interest due to their acceptance of funding from the auto, chemical, pharmaceutical, and oil industries. Not surprisingly, BCA's stance on corporate funding generated considerable controversy within the breast cancer movement, but it also facilitated new alliance building between BCA and other public health, women's rights, and environmental advocacy groups that held similar views on conflict of interest issues related to corporate philanthropy.

Democratizing the Scientific Enterprise

Barbara's push for philanthropic accountability within the breast cancer movement bolstered BCA's efforts to advance the "three Rs" of breast cancer science—relevance, rigor, and reach.[7] *Relevance* refers to whether science is asking the right questions and emphasizes underlying causes, including exposures to environmental chemicals, and assessment of the effectiveness of strategies for true prevention. *Rigor* refers to the promotion of good science—in study design, data collection, and results interpretation from research on the causes, prevention, and cure of breast cancer. *Reach* encapsulates how knowledge is disseminated to diverse audiences in the regulatory, policy, and public arenas to empower women living with breast cancer to take collective and individual action.

Barbara advanced the three Rs of breast cancer science through her constant presence at research conferences and scientific forums where new discoveries and advances in treatment regimens were presented. At these venues, she boldly pushed scientists to directly address the significance and implications of their research for women living with breast cancer. In one instance, while attending the San Antonio Breast Cancer Symposium, a presenter described how breast cancer patients were "failing treatments," and in response, during the question and answer period, Barbara deftly reminded him and the other scientists in the room that "patients don't fail treatments, treatments fail patients."[8]

Barbara also vocally challenged the mainstream cancer establishment's promotion of population-based mammography screening as an effective prevention tool, by pointing out that mammograms do not in fact *prevent* breast cancer: once screening discovers a cancerous tumor, it has not been prevented. By incessantly arguing that such prevention messages were misleading to women, Barbara and Breast Cancer Action forced other cancer organizations, such as the Susan G. Komen Foundation, to change their message on mammography screening from "early detection is the best prevention" to "early detection is the best protection." Barbara rejected this small concession as equally problematic by highlighting emerging scientific evidence that questioned the conventional wisdom about the effectiveness of mammography at saving lives, particularly for women younger than fifty. Through her writings in BCA's monthly newsletter, Barbara systematically distilled the research on this question and took the position that the benefits of mammography had been overstated and the potential harms problematically downplayed. Indeed, research now unequivocally shows that widespread mammography screening results in high false-positive rates (mistaken results indicating that a woman has cancer), as well as overdiagnosis and overtreatment (identification and treatment of cancers that are not life-threatening).

Despite the political controversy generated by its position on mammography screening among cancer groups, including the American Cancer Society, BCA took its message to women early on, and this stance has since been reaffirmed by the National Institutes of Health and the U.S. Preventive Services Task Force, which have both stated that biennial mammograms are unnecessary for women younger than fifty with average breast cancer risk.

Under Barbara's leadership, BCA worked to give women affected by breast cancer a central voice in funding decisions to support scientific research. In collaboration with other breast cancer advocacy groups and state policymakers, BCA helped to create the California Breast Cancer Research Program (CBCRP), a model initiative that supports innovative paths of inquiry to understand the causes of breast cancer. The program is funded through a cigarette tax and supports research into the causes, prevention, and cure of breast cancer as well as the challenges faced by diverse communities in accessing care for prevention and treatment of the disease. Most important, this groundbreaking research program has fundamentally shifted how funding decisions are made by ensuring that breast cancer advocates play a central role in all aspects of the scientific review process, including the initial setting of the program's research priorities and participation on review panels that evaluate the merits of funding proposals. CBCRP's governing council is required by law to include representatives of breast cancer survivor and advocacy groups.[9] Other federal research funding programs, including the Department of Defense Breast Cancer Research Program and the National Institute of Environmental Health Sciences' Breast Cancer and Environment Research Program, have subsequently emulated elements of California's initiative that engage breast cancer advocates in review panels and the scientific research. While Barbara lauded the important accomplishments of these milestone federal and California research programs, she continued to push for deeper democratization of the scientific enterprise by pointing out that as long as advocates had minority representation on review panels compared to their scientific colleagues, the potential for a paradigm shift that promoted multidisciplinary approaches to breast cancer research would not be fully realized.

Barbara's Legacy and the Road Ahead

With her deep roots in civil rights and women's rights activism, Barbara, as BCA's first full-time executive director and in collaboration with other activists, played a critical role in fundamentally transforming the breast cancer movement toward a more forward-thinking and politicized form of advocacy. This shift has yielded significant accomplishments, including a national movement that has reoriented discourse about breast cancer from an individual problem to a social and public health issue; broader public awareness about the limits of behavioral factors in explaining the steady rise in breast cancer incidence and the need to understand environmental links to the disease; and participation of women living with breast cancer in the research process. Barbara connected women's bodily experiences of breast cancer to a socioeconomic structure that exposes people to multiple environmental hazards, and she tirelessly challenged dominant scientific, medical, corporate, and political institutions as well as other breast cancer groups that emphasize treatment over prevention. While never losing sight of the importance of treatment for women living with breast cancer, Barbara insisted that reorienting activism toward true prevention compels us to understand what it is about a modern consumer society that has increased women's susceptibility to breast cancer and to demand that policymakers and scientists do more to promote the health of communities rather than simply the health of individuals.

As a leader and a mentor, Barbara inspired a new cadre of activists to carry the voices of women living with breast cancer by being outraged, skeptical optimists who continually ask the hard questions. What are the fundamental causes of this disease and how can we prevent it? How do we push scientists to undertake research that matters most to women living with breast cancer? How do we hold the medical–industrial complex accountable to ensure that it does not market unsafe and ineffective treatments to women living with or at risk for the disease? And is the traditional focus on breast cancer awareness—that is, merely *knowing* that breast cancer exists in the world around us—simply distracting us from the real work needed to end the breast cancer epidemic? This fearless engagement in the politics of breast cancer remains the core of Breast Cancer Action's mission and continues to guide its work. Under new leadership and with a larger staff, Breast Cancer Action has extended its advocacy in new directions that include pressuring state and federal legislators to improve chemicals policy by reforming the Toxic Substances Control Act and by opposing the proliferation of hydraulic fracturing ("fracking"), a process of natural gas and oil extraction that requires the intensive use of toxic chemicals, many of which are linked to breast cancer. Most important, Breast Cancer Action continues Barbara's legacy of using humor and outrage to cut through the pink noise of the breast cancer industry, telling the hard truths about this disease and ensuring that the breast cancer movement never becomes, in the words of Barbara Ehrenreich, "a lady's auxiliary to the cancer-industrial complex."[10]

Notes

1. Barbara Brenner, "Sister Support: Women Create a Breast Cancer Movement," in *Breast Cancer: Society Shapes an Epidemic*, ed. A. S. Kasper and S. J. Ferguson (New York: St. Martin's Press, 2002), 325–54.

2. S. Zavestoski, S. McCormick, and P. Brown, "Gender, Embodiment, and Disease: Environmental Breast Cancer Activists' Challenges to Science, the Biomedical Model, and Policy," *Science as Culture* 13, no. 4 (2004): 563–86.

3. L. A. G. Rie, B. A. Miller, B. F. Hankey, et al., *SEER Cancer Statistics Review, 1973–1991: Tables and Graphs*, NIH Publication no. 94-2789 (Bethesda, Md.: National Cancer Institute, 1994).

4. R. Morello-Frosch, S. Zavestoski, P. Brown, S. McCormick, B. Mayer, and R. Gasior, "Embodied Health Movements: Responses to a 'Scientized' World," in *The New Political Sociology of Science: Institutions, Networks, and Power*, ed. Kelly Moore and Scott Frickel (Madison: University of Wisconsin Press, 2006).

5. Brenner, "Sister Support."

6. J. Roemer, "Thanks, but No Thanks: Breast Cancer Group Declines Funding," *Journal of the National Cancer Institute* 91, no. 2 (1999): 108–109.

7. C. Balazs and R. Morello-Frosch, "The Three R's: How Community-Based Participatory Research Strengthens the Rigor, Relevance, and Reach of Science," *Environmental Justice* 6, no. 1 (2012): 9–16.

8. Interview by Zaylia A. Pluss for Smith College, April 20, 24, 27, 29,

and May 4, 2012, San Francisco, California. https://www.smith.edu/library/libs/ssc/oh/brenner.pdf.

9. California Health and Safety Code Section 104145. http://www.leginfo.ca.gov/cgi-bin/displaycode?section=hsc&group=104001-105000&file=104145.

10. Barbara Ehrenreich, "We Need a New Women's Health Movement," *Los Angeles Times,* December 2, 2009. http://articles.latimes.com/2009/dec/02/opinion/la-oe-ehrenreich2-2009dec02.

PART I

Building a Movement, 1995–2010

Building a Movement

Breast Cancer Action was created in 1990, and from the beginning the newsletter, published ten times a year (later quarterly), was an important part of the organization's goals. The newsletter analyzed news in the media about breast cancer, questioned drug treatments, and often challenged received opinions from the "cancer establishment," as well as connecting directly with readers and offering support and encouragement. In 1994, the number of mailing addresses was three thousand; ten years later the newsletter, now named *The Source*, went to fifteen thousand people as well as being distributed at conferences, health fairs, and in doctors' offices. By 2010, the mailing list was thirty-five thousand, and the newsletter was offered free online. BCA, now abbreviated as BCAction, is a major force in the world of breast cancer activism.

After she became the organization's executive director in 1995, Barbara Brenner's column, Letter from the Executive Editor, came out in every issue and played a significant role in uniting and inspiring the growing movement of what she called "hell-raisers" who wanted to understand breast cancer better for themselves and be part of a "thinking person's breast cancer organization." Over fifteen years, from 1996 to 2010, when she retired from Breast Cancer Action, her editorial columns were by turns thoughtful and provocative. She moved easily from dissecting drug studies and what their publicized results meant to urging action when action was necessary. The one thing all the columns had in common was the personal touch. Barbara didn't hesitate to share her own experiences as well as the humor, skepticism, and chutzpah that made her willing and able to take on the FDA, the National Cancer Institute, and other breast cancer organizations when necessary. The columns not only create a record of an important period in breast cancer movement history: they show us what health activism looks like.

Barbara had already begun writing for the newsletter in 1994 and the first piece included here is an article from 1995 (it was reprinted as a column in 2002). "Hope, Politics, and Living with Breast Cancer" summarizes well in its title and content Barbara's approach to health activism. She was always hopeful, "essentially an optimist" she called herself, and that sense of hope buoyed her politically and personally. Her idea of hope, expressed in the article and many others, wasn't faith in a "cure" or in "the end of breast cancer in twenty years." It was the hope that women affected by breast cancer could come together to demand transparency and accountability from research institutions and breast cancer organizations, and that regardless of social status and income, all women could receive honest health advice and care through every stage of their illness.

Barbara's politics came from the same source as her hope. She believed in social and economic justice, in the right of individuals and the public to get the best information and not be at the mercy of media spin and corporations that placed profit first. With her background as a lawyer and board member of the ACLU, she was alert to abuses of public trust and skeptical of entrenched power.

A case in point is her stubborn insistence on asking questions about where the money came from when it concerned groups like the Susan G. Komen Foundation; where the money went (which was often far from clear); and what result the money had (even less clear). Barbara began asking about the reasons for the proliferation of the pink ribbon as a symbol as early as 1996 in an amusing yet biting column ("Let Them Lick Stamps," August 1996) about the new U.S. Postal Service fund-raising stamp. Four years later she began questioning the trend for walking, biking, or otherwise racing for "the Cure" and traced it to the Komen Foundation ("Exercise Your Mind," March–April 2000). Barbara also used this column to look more deeply at Avon's walkathons and its marketing of pink ribbon merchandise, and to try to understand who benefited financially from the vast amounts of money raised. By September 2008, when she wrote a brief history of Breast Cancer Action's successful Think Before You Pink® campaigns ("The Organic Process of Activism: Think Before You Pink®, Then and Now," September 2008), the issue of corporate domination of the races, walks, and sales of products promoting the color pink had influenced thousands of people to respond to the way Estée Lauder, Ford Motors, Avon, and General Mills had co-opted a health epidemic to increase profits and boost their image.

Barbara's analysis of pinkwashing informs some of these columns, as does her almost annual critique of unnecessary mammograms and mammography machines as immense sources of profit for corporations. In several columns reprinted here, beginning in 1997, she takes on the misleading message pushed by some breast cancer organizations and the medical establishment that mammograms— and only mammograms—save lives ("Fiddling While Rome Burns," April–May 1997). She took it up again in a column the following year titled "Words Matter" (February–March 1998) to talk about how the language used by prominent breast cancer organizations was misleading and essentially dishonest. She parsed sentences such as "Our mission is to eradicate breast cancer through early detection" and asked bluntly "How might discovering cancer eliminate it?" She pointed out, here and elsewhere, that complacency caused by language misuse would not end the epidemic.

Her emphasis on how words matter extended to herself. In her article "Hope, Politics, and Living with Breast Cancer," Barbara discussed her own choice of what to call her illness and how to name herself. She was not a "survivor," she said, but a woman "living with breast cancer," like so many others. As she would throughout the columns over the years, she used her own experience as a touchstone. A diagnosis of breast cancer in her early forties, treated with lumpectomy, chemotherapy, and radiation, followed by a mastectomy three years later, gave her firsthand experience about what it meant to be a patient and a part of the medical system, an intimate knowledge of illness that combined with her energetic desire for justice. Barbara often invoked other women who lived with breast cancer, including her sister Nanci ("My Sister's Keeper," June–July 1998), as well as women who had died, leaving a legacy of "loss and inspiration," as she titled her first editorial column in 1996. One of the women who most inspired her was black lesbian feminist Audre Lorde, author of *The Cancer Journals* and *A Burst of Light*. "When I dare to be powerful, to use my strength in the service of my vision, then it becomes less important whether or not I am unafraid," Barbara quoted Lorde, and those words could also stand for Barbara's resolution to be strong in the face of her vision.

Over the years, the mission of Breast Cancer Action developed and clarified. The staff increased under Barbara's leadership and the newsletter expanded. Barbara occasionally paused to step back in her columns and summarize BCAction's achievements for newer readers and long-standing supporters alike. As the body of information and knowledge continued to grow, some columns repeated subjects, some were reprinted, and, thanks to the digital editions, issues mentioned in the columns could be linked to articles past and present in the newsletters.

The thirty columns reprinted here, culled from eighty or so that Barbara wrote for the newsletter over fifteen years, are representative of some of Barbara's strongest writing and abiding concerns. Here she dispensed information, analyzed medical trials, took corporations to task, and continued to hold other breast cancer organizations accountable for how they raised their funds and how they spent those funds. Here, too, with humor and more than a touch of outrageousness, she told of some of her adventures at conferences and in meetings and never hesitated to show her irritation at the annual folly of Breast Cancer Awareness Month—or "October Madness Redux," as she once called it.

Her columns and the newsletters were read by thousands of people eager for substantial information on their disease. Her calls for action brought tangible results and caused her readers to become more skeptical and smarter about claims made by researchers and advertisers alike. Barbara also offered hope in these columns—not only about living with breast cancer, but a deeper and more expansive sense of hope—for dignity, integrity, and social justice.

A Note on Science, Sources, and Further Resources

Barbara Brenner was an extraordinary health activist. She came to breast cancer and Breast Cancer Action from a background in the social sciences, public policy, and the law, from which she drew skills in research, analysis, and advocacy. As she emerged into the world of health activism, she applied these skills to decoding the language of scientific research on breast cancer and ALS. She then presented and criticized data and methodology in her speeches and writings for the general public. Although she was not a trained medical research scientist, Barbara formulated critiques of such issues as mammogram screening and clinical trials. These critiques appeared not only in her columns and blog posts but as topical informational articles in the newsletter from 1995 to 2010. Eventually many of these ideas became part of BCAction's public platform, as guidelines and fact sheets, in print and online at the website; videos and webinars followed.

The science that Barbara writes about in her columns and posts was based on information available at the time from a variety of sources. Over the past twenty years some of the positions held by BCAction have evolved, and not only for BCAction but also for other organizations. Readers interested in the current aspects of breast cancer research may find more updated information as well as BCAction's positions and suggestions on the website, www.bcaction. org. Many of the back issues of *The Source* (previously called the *BCA Newsletter*) have been digitized, offering links to columns of Barbara's that weren't included in this collection as well as other articles. In editing this collection, especially the blog posts, I've retained some links that are still live and removed others. The scientific research as Barbara understood it is presented as she wrote it.

Hope, Politics, and Living with Breast Cancer

I spend many hours a week communicating across cyberspace with other people concerned about breast cancer. In a recent exchange with Internet colleagues, I posed the question of what those of us who have been treated for breast cancer should call ourselves. The discussion raised important questions about the relationship between hope and politics.

I do not call myself a breast cancer survivor, nor do I refer to others who have been diagnosed with breast cancer as survivors. The term suggests to the world—wrongly—that breast cancer is curable. It is true, thank goodness, that many of us will live long enough to die of something else. But no one who has been diagnosed with invasive breast cancer can ever say truthfully that the cancer will not recur.

For me, the term *survivor* also carries a notion that I am not dead of breast cancer because I am somehow better or different from the hundreds of thousands of women who have died of the disease.

I have found no single word that conveys what I would like to convey when I speak of my experience with breast cancer: that it has changed my life permanently and in many ways, whether the cancer kills me or not. The phrase "living with breast cancer" is one option. It tells others that it is possible to live with this disease, while acknowledging implicitly that not all of us are so lucky. It also communicates in a small way that the diagnosis is a life-transforming event. But it suggests (as would the phrase "I have breast cancer") that the person referred to is currently in treatment or in need of treatment. And because of the common use of the term "living with AIDS," it implies that women with breast cancer will die of the disease, unless something else kills them first.

When I sent these ideas to my online breast cancer group, one person objected to the phrase "living with breast cancer" because it echoed for her the American Cancer Society's Living with Cancer program, which, for her, is a campaign of false hope and fear. This woman wanted to focus attention on the need to prevent breast cancer. Another member of the group wondered in response whether we must sacrifice hope in order to bring the necessary political pressure to bear to find cures and preventive measures.

Hope is defined in the *American College Dictionary* as "the expectation of something desired," or "confidence in a future event." At this moment, any expectation or confidence that breast cancer, once treated, will never recur is indeed a false hope. There is no cure for breast cancer. Do we need to make people believe that there is a cure because otherwise people will feel helpless in the face of a diagnosis? Conversely, do we need to make people understand that there is no cure if we are ever to expect sufficient attention to be paid to the breast cancer epidemic?

These questions highlight for me the place where the personal and the political—which I generally take to be one and the same—part company. People who are ill, and those who love them, need hope. They need to believe that they or their loved ones may be cured because, in fact, some of them will be, and because hope is essential to the human spirit. In fact, sometimes after a person has finished treatment, and for no reason that anyone can identify, the cancer may not recur. But the same treatment given to another woman or thousands of other women cannot be guaranteed to cure any of those people. And it is this fact that must propel political action, and that makes the work of BCA so important.

As long as people pretend that there is a cure for breast cancer, women will continue to die from neglect of this disease. Two million women in the United States are living day in and day out with the possibility of a recurrence of breast cancer. People must understand this reality if effective pressure is to be brought to bear on governmental, scientific, and medical institutions to find effective ways of ending this epidemic.

Polio was considered a public health crisis when 50,000 people became ill with (and 3,300 died of) the disease in one year. What will it take for breast cancer to get the same kind of attention?

It will take women who have been diagnosed and those at risk (which is, after all, all women) making themselves heard about the need for cure and prevention. So—because the personal is political—to anyone who cares to know and many who don't, I am a woman living with breast cancer.

August 1995

Loss and Inspiration

Educating the world about breast cancer is often about statistics: how many people are diagnosed each day? How many die? What percentage carries the breast cancer gene? What are the chances of surviving? How many pesticides are used on our food, and how do they affect us?

But the numbers only tell a part of the story. Behind each number is a woman, connected to other human beings and contributing to the world, until her death leaves a gaping hole in the fabric of the universe. Too often, we emphasize the numbers instead of the people. I'd like to tell you about two women who died recently from breast cancer. Their lives contain lessons for all of us.

Pat Anesi was a teacher of English as a second language (ESL), most recently and for many years at San Francisco City College. I first learned about Pat when BCA started receiving contributions in her memory. We get far too many gifts like this, but the ones for Pat were remarkable in that many of them came in very small amounts or from distant shores, with notes from her former students.

I was intrigued by the outpouring of love for Pat Anesi, so I set out to learn more about her. Months after her death, her colleagues at City College still cried when they talked about what Pat had meant to them. She was a devoted teacher who loved her work and felt lucky to be able to do it in a creative way.

Pat made it a point to bring the outside world into her classroom. She was one of the first to use film and video in an ESL class. She initiated the computer lab for ESL students at City College, creating a program that helped the students cross the bridge between ESL work and computer classes in English. Pat connected with her students by doing things with them outside of the classroom and staying in touch long after they had left the ESL program. A dear friend and colleague told me that Pat did three times as much as other teachers. Her students responded to that commitment.

Besides being a dedicated teacher, Pat Anesi was fun. She appreciated life's absurdities and had a wonderful sense of humor. She loved mystery books and wearing '40s style hats and going to "tea" with her friends. She was a proud and private person, a devoted and loving daughter and sister, and the kind of friend who would never let you down.

First diagnosed with breast cancer about three years ago, Pat never spoke of it. When friends learned of her illness, it struck them as ironic that Pat, who always took such good care of herself physically, would be the one among them confronting breast cancer. As her illness advanced, Pat spoke more openly about her feelings about it. She was appalled by how crude the treatments were. Her friends were impressed by her valiance and her consideration of others, even in the face of her own illness.

When Pat Anesi died in October 1995 at age fifty-one, she left behind her sister, many longtime friends, and hundreds of students who miss her creativity, her loyalty, her devotion to education, her strong opinions, and her sense of humor. She asked her friends to contribute to BCA because she believed that our work makes a difference.

On the other side of the country, Karen Caviglia was a computer software engineer, writer, and political activist living in Shrewsbury, Massachusetts. She was diagnosed with breast cancer in 1988, but the disease had been a presence in her life long before her own diagnosis. Her grandmother died of breast cancer, her mother has been living with the disease for eighteen years, and her mother-in-law struggled with metastatic disease for ten years as a single mother of three working on a PhD in English.

I "met" Karen online when she posted a message in response to one about a fashion show for "breast cancer survivors." Karen was outraged at the attempts to put a pretty face on this disease. The political

kinship I felt with her across cyberspace became the basis of a regular
e-mail correspondence that Karen and I carried on for many months,
until I became too busy and she too ill.

But even in the midst of her struggle with metastatic breast
cancer, Karen found the energy to communicate with me about this
newsletter and to encourage BCA's work. It was through BCA that
Karen learned about HER2/neu, the treatment she was on (as part of
the trial) when she died. And she saw BCA as a model for work that
she was doing in Massachusetts. She was a founding member of the
Massachusetts Breast Cancer Coalition and the National Breast Cancer Coalition, as well as a member of BCA.

But Karen's life was about far more than breast cancer. She was
active on many fronts, believing that the world is an "interconnected
web," and that none of us is safe until all of us are safe. People who
knew her describe her as totally honest, articulate, extraordinarily
intelligent, focused and funny, brave and noble. She held three master's degrees, was an active member of her church, a loving daughter,
mother, partner, and aunt, and continued as much as possible to live
life to its fullest even as breast cancer sapped her strength. Less than
six months before her death, she swam a mile in Walden Pond as part
of Against the Tide, a fund-raiser for breast cancer research in Massachusetts. She inspired others. As one of her e-mail buddies wrote,
"Karen Caviglia walked boldly in the shadows where my fears lurk.
Her footsteps resound in my heart. With honesty and strength, she
gave substance to my hope that life can remain rich in the face of
advanced breast cancer."

Reflecting on her past and her future, Karen said, "I always suspected that I would get old and have breast cancer. I was half right."
Karen died on January 5, 1996. Like Pat Anesi, she was fifty-one
years old.

Karen Caviglia once wrote that she carried the stories of midlife
women in her heart as a fuel supply for the anger she needed to keep
fighting the epidemic. Audre Lorde, who died of breast cancer at age
fifty-eight, captured the essence of the struggle: "As warriors our job
is to actively and consciously survive [cancer] for as long as possible,
remembering that in order to win, the aggressor must conquer, but
the resisters need only survive. Our battle is to define survival in ways

that are acceptable and nourishing to us, meaning with substance and style. Substance. Our work. Style. True to ourselves." Pat Anesi and Karen Caviglia survived with substance and style. They succumbed in the primes of their lives, surrendering nothing of who they were. They are two of the women whose lives and deaths fuel the work of BCA. They are some of the people behind the numbers. We will not forget them.

April 1996

✿

Let Them Lick Stamps

In a culture where television actors portraying hemorrhoid sufferers are all smiles, it should come as no surprise that we now have a stamp that touts breast cancer awareness without communicating anything about the disease. Issued in conjunction with the Susan G. Komen Foundation's 1996 Race for the Cure in Washington, D.C., the stamp portrays the bare shoulder of a young, beautifully coiffed white woman, seen from the back. A pink ribbon is shown in the lower right corner. If the stamp didn't say "Breast Cancer Awareness" along the edge, most people would no doubt conclude that the stamp commemorates either women's hair fashion or shoulder surgery.

I guess it would be too radical to portray an actual woman's breast on a postage stamp, and certainly stamps glorifying empty symbols are nothing new. But I find this stamp particularly offensive in the way it combines a clichéd image of an unclothed woman with the pink ribbon symbol that does nothing to bring attention to what is really needed to end the breast cancer epidemic. A stamp that would accomplish that purpose would need to look more like the stamp BCA would prefer, depicting symbolic breasts and environmental hazards.

Think for a moment about what the Postal Service stamp shows. It is true that alarming numbers of young women do get breast cancer, but they do not end up for the most part modeling their lovely young bodies. They far too often end up dead: breast cancer is the most common cause of death for women between the ages of thirty-five and fifty-four. If the stamp is intended to remind women to get mammograms, as the Komen Race does, it should depict the women for whom they may do the most good—older women and African Americans.

And then there's the pink ribbon. I'm not certain how a pink ribbon came to be a breast cancer symbol. First there was the yellow ribbon, meant to bring American hostages home from Iran. Then the red ribbon began appearing on the lapels of Hollywood stars as a way of bringing attention to the devastation that AIDS had wrought (and continues to wreak) on the entertainment community. When people started noticing that there was an awful lot of breast cancer around, someone apparently came up with the idea of quietly and gently raising consciousness about the disease by pastel-coloring a symbol copied from the AIDS movement.

The first ribbons were of pink cloth. Now you can get them in cloisonné or enameled and trimmed in gold, or studded with diamonds, or on your postage stamps. But what do they tell the world about breast cancer? This is not a pastel-colored disease, and little strips of cloth will not end the epidemic.

The stamp was released with great public fanfare at post offices throughout the country. In San Francisco, the head of the breast clinic at San Francisco General Hospital appeared at the press conference declaring that the stamp honors, among others, "those who can prevent [breast cancer] through proper screening." If doctors treating breast cancer can't tell the difference between prevention and detection, is it any wonder that the rest of the world can't? After all, the American Cancer Society and the Susan G. Komen Foundation have for years promoted mammograms as your best prevention. Anyone who thinks about it for ten seconds recognizes that mammograms don't prevent breast cancer. And those who investigate the matter even a little bit will learn that mammograms don't even detect breast cancer in a large number of cases.

Don't get me wrong. I believe that raising awareness of breast cancer is critical to ending the epidemic. But the awareness that will motivate change is awareness about the realities of this dreaded disease. It's not about pretty bare shoulders and pink ribbons.

So the symbol I wear—besides the scars and radiation tattoos on my left breast—is the one that appears on our Prayer Flags and on BCA's version of a breast cancer awareness stamp. The symbol is an artistic interpretation of a coil that symbolized the full moon to an ancient Maltese matriarchal society. That culture believed that the lunar cycle was a cycle of rejuvenation, and its women warriors carried the symbol of the moon on breastplates that they wore into battle. I wear that symbol now—embossed in gold color on a deep purple background—as part of the battle I wage every day against breast cancer. So I don't wear pink ribbons and I won't be buying any of the new breast cancer awareness stamps. I don't have time for empty symbols.

August–September 1996

Fiddling While Rome Burns

The Latest Mammogram Controversy

Unless you were in a media blackout, you could hardly miss it. The National Institutes of Health (NIH) held a consensus development conference in January on mammography screening for women aged forty to forty-nine. The conclusions reached by the panel have generated extensive comment. The general impression conveyed by the press is that women are outraged by the failure of the conference to recommend regular mammograms for women in their forties.[1]

The debate raises a number of issues.

First, why were people expecting the panel to make a recommendation for regular screening? The media strongly indicated before the conference began that the only reasonable conclusion would be a renewed recommendation[2] that women begin regular screening at age forty.[3] This press view almost certainly reflects the influence of the National Cancer Institute (NCI) and the American Cancer Society (ACS) on how the media covers and how the public perceives cancer issues. Dr. Richard Klausner, director of the NCI, who convened the conference, said afterward that his own view is that there is a net benefit from screening of women aged forty to forty-nine.[4]

Mammograms have been the centerpiece of the ACS's campaign against breast cancer since 1983.[5] As part of that campaign, the ACS has been advising women aged forty to forty-nine to have regular mammograms, despite the lack of agreement on the benefits of the procedure. Following the NIH conference, the ACS restated its support of mammograms every one to two years for women forty to forty-nine.[6] The ACS is so locked into the "mammograms are your best protection" message of "breast health" that, by the time you read this column, it will have held its own conference in March to consider whether to recommend annual mammograms for women in this age group. (Dollars to donuts, I'm betting they answer the question with a resounding "yes.")

Despite the pressure to find clear benefits justifying a recommendation of regular screening mammograms for women forty to forty-nine, the NIH panel concluded that the scientific evidence does not support such a recommendation. Instead, the panel stated: "At the present time, the available data do not warrant a single recommendation for mammography for all women in their forties. Each woman should decide for herself whether to undergo mammography. . . . [A] woman should have access to the best possible information in an understandable and usable form. Her health care provider must be equipped with sufficient information to facilitate her decision-making process. . . . [C]osts of mammograms should be reimbursed by third-party payers or covered by health maintenance organizations."[7]

By itself, this statement is hardly controversial. After all, it argues—as does BCA's Policy on Mammography—for informed decision making by women faced with conflicting data about the benefits of the technology. Which brings me to the second issue that the debate highlights: why all the outrage about the recommendations?

The short answer to this question lies in the way the media likes to cover stories. Personal testimonials by women who believe their lives have been saved by mammograms make much better and more compelling reading than the text of the consensus conference's report. Controversy also makes better press. In the *New York Times*, the story was presented as a conflict pitting radiologists and breast cancer patients against public health specialists and some feminists.[8]

Then, of course, there are those whose vested interests impassion their arguments. Dr. Michael Linver, director of mammography at X-Ray Associates of New Mexico and a presenter at the conference, commented on the findings: "I do fear that this is tantamount to a death sentence [for women in their forties]. I grieve for them."[9] The American College of Radiology, whose members make part of their livings by doing mammograms, not only criticized the consensus statement but recommended that the screening interval for women forty to forty-nine be shortened to once a year. Let's see, now: that's twice as many mammograms, which means twice as much income, right?

And there is the ACS, which found it "especially troubling that the panel would issue a pessimistic statement, and conclude once again that the burden of decision for a woman in her forties is hers alone."[10] Of course, none of the conclusions would trouble the ACS if the organization had been more forthcoming in the first instance about the risks and benefits of mammographic screening. By promoting mammograms as an unqualified good, the ACS has helped to mislead American women about the value of the technology.[11]

The debate ignores the third and most fundamental problem. If there is any reason for outrage, it is this: as long as we are spending our time, energy, and money on the mammogram debate, we are distracted from finding a non–radiation-based detection method that works, discovering effective treatments, and offering primary prevention. Just as Nero fiddled while Rome burned, we are spending enormous resources on an aspect of breast cancer that ultimately does very little, if anything, to save lives.

Reverberations from the recommendations demonstrate this misguided effort. Dr. Klausner was so unhappy with the conclusion of the consensus panel that he spent more taxpayer money to convene the National Cancer Advisory Board (NCAB) in February 1997 to review the decision. What we might expect from those deliberations is revealed by the comments of one member of the NCAB who has publicly stated that Klausner's actions "constitute a moral stand and a courageous stand" and prove that Klausner "cares about the health of American women."[12]

The panel's report itself includes some of the same misguided research recommendations that keep us from learning what causes and what prevents breast cancer. As to directions for future study, the panel identifies eighteen research questions that need to be answered. All of them concern the utility and value of mammograms. When will we stop spending money on a technology that gains us so little in terms of reducing the death rate from breast cancer? Take the call for a study of the effectiveness of mammography for African American women. It's a waste of valuable resources unless it helps resolve more important questions, such as why African American women, who develop the disease less often, die more often and sooner than white women.

Too much attention is being focused on the mammography debate and away from the real questions that need to be answered. The interests that benefit while our efforts are diverted from the hard issues of the breast cancer epidemic are legion. None of us can afford to allow them to prevail. After all, Rome is burning.

April–May 1997

Notes

1. See "Mammogram Panel Only Adds to Furor," *USA Today*, January 24-26, 1997; "Stand on Mammograms Greeted by Outrage," *New York Times*, January 28, 1997.

2. Since 1983, the American Cancer Society (ACS) has recommended that women forty to forty-nine have screening mammograms every one to two years. The National Cancer Institute (NCI) began making the same recommendation in 1987. In 1993, the NCI decided that the scientific evidence did not support this recommendation and withdrew it. The ACS and many other cancer organizations disagreed and continued to urge regular screening mammograms for women in this age group.

3. See "Personal Health: New Studies Indicate That Women in Their 40s Benefit from Annual Mammograms," *New York Times*, December 4, 1996; "News You Can Use: The Great Mammogram Debate," *U.S. News and World Report*, January 27, 1997.

4. "Mammogram Talks Prove Indefinite," *New York Times*, January 24, 1997.

5. S. Batt, *Patient No More: The Politics of Breast Cancer* (Charlottetown, P.E.I., Canada: Gynergy Books, 1994), 41.

6. "NIH Statement Doesn't Resolve Mammography Controversy," *The Cancer Letter* 23, no. 4 (January 31, 1997).

7. National Institutes of Health Consensus Development Conference Statement, "Breast Cancer Screening for Women Ages 40–49," January 21–23, 1997.

8. "Mammograms for Women in 40s Debated by Experts," *New York Times*, January 22, 1997.

9. "Mammogram Talks Prove Indefinite."

10. "NIH Statement Doesn't Resolve Mammography Controversy."

11. See "Mammography under Fire," *BCA Newsletter*, no. 38 (October/November 1996). See also Batt, *Patient No More*, 243.

12. Ellen Sigal, member of NCAB, quoted in *BCA Newsletter*, "Mammography Screening for Ages 40–49 Not Supported by Data, NIH Panel Says," *The Cancer Letter* 23, no. 4 (January 31, 1997). The implication that the consensus panel is indifferent to the health of American women is bad enough. What is worse is Ms. Sigal's suggestion that continuing to focus on the issue of mammograms for forty- to forty-nine-year-olds somehow puts the NCI director on the cutting edge of the efforts to end the breast cancer epidemic.

Reflections on a Handmaid's Tale

The first thing I do after showering in the morning is read the newspaper—two of them, in fact. As I eat breakfast, I listen to radio news. At night, before I go to sleep, I watch the late-night news. Like the hapless protagonist in Margaret Atwood's 1986 novel *The Handmaid's Tale*, "I'm ravenous for news, any kind of news; even if it's false news, it must mean something."[1] And the first thing I look for is breast cancer stories.

While my attention usually focuses on the particular story that has caught the media's eye, recent news items have led me to take a step back and ponder the bigger picture. In particular, stories about the link between abortion and breast cancer risk and a story about San Francisco Bay Area breast cancer risk factors suggest that we need to think about the underlying message that studies and stories like these send: that women have abandoned their proper roles as mothers and homemakers, and that their health requires that they step back into those roles.

The abortion story is pretty obvious. The heated political debate about abortion rights in the United States has led the contestants in that battle to look for any evidence to support their view. Thus, despite the absence of any study that reliably establishes a link between abortion and breast cancer,[2] abortion opponents point to breast cancer risk as a reason not to terminate a pregnancy.[3] The message here is clear: women should have babies, not abortions.

The other "risk factor" studies are more insidious, but the message is the same. In July, the National Cancer Institute published a study titled "Regional Differences in Known Risk Factors and the

Higher Incidence of Breast Cancer in San Francisco."[4] The authors of the study looked at some of the known and probable risk factors for breast cancer and concluded that the record-high levels of breast cancer in the Bay Area are explained by those factors. The factors examined were parity (whether the woman has given birth to a child), age at first full-term pregnancy, breastfeeding, age at menarche (when menstruation began), age at menopause, and alcohol consumption.

Of course, other than when we start and stop menstruating, all of these risk factors have to do with behavior: whether and when we have children, whether we breastfeed our children, whether we drink alcohol. And—surprise, surprise—all of these behavioral factors cut in the same direction. So one message here is that breast cancer rates will decline when more women become teetotaling, breastfeeding young mothers.

But there is another message as well. As the principal author of the study says, "We want women in the Bay Area to know that this environment is not causing more breast cancer."[5] That's a very bold conclusion from a study that did not examine environmental factors. The known risk factors for breast cancer at best explain only 30 percent to 40 percent of all cases of the disease. So why do the study's authors want us to conclude that the increased incidence of breast cancer over the past thirty years (from a lifetime risk of one in twenty to one in eight) is not related to environment? Why do they focus instead on factors we can individually "control"?

Might it be that if we believe our individual behavior is causing breast cancer, we won't press for changes in "business as usual"? Might it be that encouraging women to retreat from the workplace to the nursery is part of a larger backlash against the growing choices women have in their lives?

Which brings me back to *The Handmaid's Tale.* In that book, the world has been so devastated by environmental contamination that birth rates have fallen precipitously. Members of the political and economic elite in the nation of Gilead are given handmaids whose sole function is to serve as surrogate mothers, and the handmaids are prohibited from putting their reproductive capacity at risk. What led to Gilead's predicament, the protagonist notes, is that, in days gone by, women seemed to be able to choose. The people in power were threatened by individuals having too much choice. The changes that led to the handmaid's plight in Atwood's chilling novel did not arise overnight. "Nothing changes instantaneously: in a gradually heating bathtub you'd be boiled to death before you knew it." We should all be watching the temperature gauge and working to moderate the heat. We need to pay close attention to the underlying messages and to challenge them. When the study reported is about things we already know, it's a good bet there is something more—and more insidious—than meets the eye.

October–November 1997

Notes

1. Margaret Atwood, *The Handmaid's Tale* (Boston: Houghton Mifflin, 1986).

2. Mads Melbye, Jan Wohlfahrt, Jørgen H. Olsen, et al., "Induced Abortion and the Risk of Breast Cancer," *New England Journal of Medicine* 336 (January 9, 1997): 81–85.

3. J. Brind, V. M. Chinchilli, W. B. Severs, and J. Summy-Long, "Induced Abortion as an Independent Risk Factor for Breast Cancer: A Comprehensive Review and Meta-analysis," *Journal of Epidemiological and Community Health* 50 (October 15, 1996): 481–96. This study was funded by the Pennsylvania state legislature, one of the most antiabortion legislatures in the United States.

4. A. S. Robbins, S. Brescianini, and J. L. Kelsey, "Regional Differences in Known Risk Factors and the Higher Incidence of Breast Cancer in San Francisco," *Journal of the National Cancer Institute* 89 (13): 960–65.

5. Teresa Moore, "Bay Area Cancer Rates Interpreted: Late Childbearing Raises Risk for White Women," *San Francisco Chronicle*, July 3, 1997.

Words Matter

Every once in a while I'm reminded of some basic principles in community education and organizing. One of these principles was perhaps made most familiar to us by Dr. Seuss's Horton the Elephant, whose mantra was, "I meant what I said, and I said what I meant." Or, more succinctly: words matter. I've recently been reminded of why and how much they matter.

A daylong meeting of representatives of various California breast cancer organizations began with self-introductions. Three of the people in the room represented different chapters of the Susan G. Komen Breast Cancer Foundation. One person spoke for all three when she said, "Our mission is to eradicate breast cancer through early detection." I almost fell off my chair trying to make sense of that statement.

"Eradicate" means to eliminate. "Detection" is the act of discovering. How might discovering cancer eliminate it? The two words "eradicate" and "detection" cannot rationally be used together in the same sentence, at least not when breast cancer is the subject of the sentence. To eradicate breast cancer, we will have to prevent it. Prevention is not the same as detection. While early detection is an admirable and important goal (after all, the chances of long-term survival are far better if breast cancer is found "early"), it has nothing to do with eliminating the disease.

Not so long ago, groups like the Komen Foundation touted mammograms (to date the best available tool for early detection) as "your best prevention." While cancer charities have stopped using this phrase, the "eradication through early detection" message is not very different. These messages have had a significant impact: people still think of mammograms as prevention.

A highly educated friend of mine recently questioned my statement about the lack of any known way to prevent breast cancer by asking me, "But what about mammograms?" I have no reason to believe that the general public is any better informed on the issue of breast cancer prevention than my friend is.

Experience tells me that the public is similarly ill-informed about the concept of a cure. So many people have heard the October mantra (promoted by Zeneca Corporation, the Centers for Disease Control, the American Cancer Society, and other cancer charities) that "breast cancer found early is almost 100 percent curable" that there is now a widespread belief that breast cancer can be cured. But what "almost 100 percent curable" actually means is that women whose breast cancer is found first on a mammogram have a 92 percent to 95 percent chance of being alive (though not necessarily disease-free) five years after diagnosis. The difference between that definition and "cure" (being restored to a normal life expectancy) is vast indeed. How vast can be seen from the ten-year survival rate (67.1 percent for women diagnosed in 1984) and the twenty-year survival rate (51.4 percent for women diagnosed in 1974). (Source: *SEER Cancer Statistics Review, 1973–1994*.)

And it can also be seen in the terror that invades our lives and those of our loved ones every time a doctor tells us that something seems not quite right and we need some additional diagnostic test to check for evidence of metastasis. In December, I was breathless for a day while awaiting the results of a chest X-ray taken after a "routine" follow-up appointment with my surgeon. If surgery, radiation, and chemotherapy cured me, why would my doctor be worried about metastasis, and why would I be terrified by the words, "I think you should have a chest X-ray"?

So words matter. They matter because people are far less likely to take action when they believe that a problem has been resolved. People who believe that mammograms prevent breast cancer or that breast cancer detected early can be cured are far less likely to be aggressive about their own health care or highly engaged in the work that needs to be done to end the breast cancer epidemic.

Words matter because they can lead to complacency, and complacency will not end this epidemic. So the next time you hear or see the words "early detection" and "prevention" or "eradication" in the same sentence, ask the speaker/writer what he or she means and correct any misinformation. And the next time you notice the words "cure" and "breast cancer" together, correct the record. Finding true prevention and a real cure depend on it.

February–March 1998

My Sister's Keeper

Like most women with breast cancer, I often receive calls from friends and acquaintances of friends who have just been diagnosed with the disease. I recently received one of those calls from someone I had hoped would never need such help—my younger sister, Nanci. As I write this column, three weeks after Nanci's mastectomy, she's doing as well as can be expected, healing physically and struggling to adjust to having been drafted into the army of one-breasted women. Nanci's experience is instructive on so many levels that I've asked her if I could describe it in this column.

The first hint of a problem came as the result of a routine mammogram. Nanci, who is now forty-three years old, has been having annual mammograms since my diagnosis at age forty-one in 1993. Following this year's X-ray, Nanci got a call from the radiology center asking her to come back for more pictures. How many of us have been in this place? But since I knew there was a good chance of a false positive (most recently highlighted in a *New England Journal of Medicine* report; see "Study Finds High Rate of Mammogram False Alarms," *San Francisco Chronicle*, April 16, 1998), especially for someone so young, I was reassuring.

When Nanci went in for her follow-up, she had an ultrasound exam. The technician showed her clusters of microcalcifications and explained that these clusters had prompted the callback. When Nanci met later with the radiologist, he suggested that she wait six months and then have another mammogram. While he did not explain to her what he was concerned about, he did say that he would consult with his chief of staff about the appropriateness of his recommendation.

Maybe because we were brought up in the same household, Nanci refused to take the "wait and see" advice. When we talked, she expressed great discomfort with the radiologist's approach and said that she thought she should see a breast surgeon. By the time Nanci finally received the written report from the radiologist so she could see the surgeon, she was pretty stressed out. Her surgeon examined the mammogram and ultrasound results, took some of his own mammograms, and told Nanci that the clusters of microcalcifications—three in all—needed to come out. This was the only way to tell for sure whether she was facing breast cancer. Core biopsies were not an option because of the number of sites. Excisional biopsies were needed.

Because the lesions in her right breast could not be felt, wire localizations were necessary to assure that the correct tissue was biopsied. After enduring the excruciating process of having three wires placed in her breast, Nanci underwent the biopsy surgery. Two days later, Nanci received a call from the doctor's office, asking her to come in at 9 o'clock that night. She knew the news would not be good.

Nanci called me after she returned from her doctor's office, with notes about her conversation with the surgeon. The biopsies had revealed DCIS (ductal carcinoma in situ) in two places in her breast. There were no clear margins. The nuclear grade was II/III. (Tumors are graded from one to three or four, with higher numbers indicating a more aggressive disease.) The doctor believed that Nanci needed a mastectomy. She was upset and terrified but knew what she needed to do.

We talked at length about what DCIS is, about mastectomy surgery, and about immediate reconstructive surgery, which her surgeon was suggesting but which Nanci was not inclined to do. I encouraged her to seek a second opinion, but Nanci trusted her surgeon and felt strongly that his mastectomy recommendation was right for her.

We spoke every day by phone as Nanci came to grips with what she was facing. She visited a store that specializes in breast prostheses and resolved not to have reconstruction. She called on her terrific husband and wonderful friends to be with her at critical times. She was sad and strong. And she was a nervous wreck, unable to get more than a few hours of sleep at a time.

Nanci decided to have her mastectomy as an outpatient (she

hates hospitals), and I went east to be with her. I watched her family and friends rally around to take care of her. I was once again impressed by who my sister Nanci is, how she has built her community, and how the difficult choices around a breast cancer diagnosis must ultimately be made alone.

I was unhappily impressed by a couple of other things. Nanci lives in a major metropolitan center in Baltimore. She received her mammogram and the "wait and see" advice at one of the leading medical complexes in the region. Why, in 1998, was it necessary for my sister to write to the radiologist to alert him to the dangers to which his advice exposed her and to call on him to change the way he treats women?

And while I waited to hear from Nanci about her postbiopsy visit to the surgeon, the National Cancer Institute and the American Cancer Society were proudly announcing the latest figures on incidence and mortality. But those figures do not include DCIS. When you read all the fine print in the reports, you find that the expected 36,900 cases of DCIS are in addition to the estimated 180,300 new cases of breast cancer this year in the United States.

But Nanci's experience is the experience of breast cancer. She has faced the terror of diagnosis and is coping with the effects of treatment. So why are these cases excluded from the statistics? Is it because DCIS is not life-threatening? Or is it because when added to the cases of invasive breast cancer the DCIS numbers put us frighteningly above 200,000 cases of breast cancer a year? As the invasive cancer numbers go down, the DCIS numbers go up. When screening mammograms reduce mortality, they do so largely by finding breast cancer before it becomes invasive. But taking the invasive and the in situ cases together, the number of breast cancer cases increased by 1,500 from 1996 to 1998. Behind each of these numbers is a story like Nanci's.

Clearly, we have much work to do. I am so sorry that my sister has been dragged into the world of breast cancer, but I am thrilled that her prognosis is excellent and happy to have her join activists working to save future generations from the cancer epidemic.

June–July 1998

Educate, Agitate, Organize—Now!

When I dare to be powerful, to use my strength in the service of my vision, then it becomes less important whether or not I am unafraid.

—AUDRE LORDE, *THE CANCER JOURNALS*

People sometimes ask me how Breast Cancer Action is different from other breast cancer organizations. Our newly revised mission statement captures it: BCA carries the voices of people affected by breast cancer to inspire and compel the changes necessary to end the breast cancer epidemic. But if I don't have time to recite this, I simply say, "We're the hell-raisers." So it is particularly fitting that our Second Annual Town Meeting will feature three mighty women, each of whom is a hell-raiser in her own right, and each of whom has a deep personal connection to what I have come to refer to as "the dreaded sisterhood" of women living with breast cancer. Author/activist Dorothy Allison witnessed her mother's breast cancer experience. Poet/essayist/activist June Jordan has written and spoken passionately and eloquently about her own diagnosis and treatment. And author/cultural commentator Anne Lamott lost her best friend to breast cancer. It's hard for me to imagine a more powerful afternoon than one spent in the company of these three women, talking about how each of us can do something to help end this epidemic.

The clarion call to action that will ring from this town meeting will resonate with everyone whose life has been touched by breast cancer. And whose hasn't? If you are reading this newsletter, you almost certainly know people who have been diagnosed. You may well have known people whose lives were cut short by the disease. And you and your friends may wonder what you can do that might make a difference. If so, this town meeting is for you and for everyone you care about.

Our five task forces—Community Outreach, Action Alert, Legislative Action, Media Response, and Treatment Issues—are giving people something to do, something that makes a real difference. We know how busy everyone is, so to join a task force you don't have to sign your life away. We ask that you make a commitment to do three things over the next year—whether it's write three letters to your local newspaper, or contact three organizations or groups that need to hear about what is really happening in breast cancer, or attend three demonstrations against the latest environmental outrage. At the town meeting, you will learn more about the task forces and have a chance to get involved in one or more of them.

One of the things that we will do at the town meeting is rename the Action Alert Task Force as the Audre Lorde Action Brigade. Not long after I was diagnosed with breast cancer in 1993, friends suggested that I read some of Audre Lorde's writings about her experience with the disease. That reading—particularly of *The Cancer Journals* and *A Burst of Light*—inspired me to become a breast cancer activist. The passion of Audre Lorde's words and the clarity of her vision continue to inspire my activism and, in many ways, the work of BCA. It was Lorde who said, "While we fortify ourselves with visions of the future, we must arm ourselves with accurate perceptions of the barriers between us and that future." At our Second Annual Town Meeting we will do both. I hope to see you there.

August–September 1998

One Pill Makes You Smaller . . .

A number of things that crossed my desk in the past few months have made me think that we are all living in a world as out of kilter as Alice's Wonderland.

Most of them have to do with the search for the patentable drug that will protect women from breast cancer. And it seems that women are being made the unwitting guinea pigs in the effort. What else are we to think when Larry Norton, director of the breast center at Memorial Sloan Kettering Cancer Center in New York, is quoted in *Ob/Gyn News* as saying that "almost all postmenopausal women in the United States will be receiving a drug shortly to improve their health and lower their odds of getting breast cancer"? (See "Tamoxifen Prevents Breast Cancer, but Questions Remain," *Ob/Gyn News*, May 1, 1998.) Dr. Norton's statement was made with regard to raloxifene, and he is one of the principal investigators of a major study of the drug. Raloxifene is a selective estrogen response modifier, or SERM, that is closely related to tamoxifen, manufactured by Eli Lilly under the trademark Evista. It's probably not that astonishing to learn that Dr. Norton is a paid consultant to Eli Lilly.

Surely, though, a reasonable sense of proportion is missing when the announcement of the results of the Breast Cancer Prevention Trial (BCPT-1) by the National Cancer Institute (NCI) sparks an avalanche of media coverage, while the *Lancet's* publication of the preliminary results of two European trials is met with a deafening silence. The non-U.S. trials of healthy women at high risk for breast cancer did not show that tamoxifen had any significant preventative effect. (The *New York Times*, which reported extensively on the NCI's

BCPT-1, did not even mention the European studies in the West Coast edition of the paper. Those whose newspaper of choice is the *Times* will have missed out on the new information that undermines the initial reports about tamoxifen for healthy women. (Not surprising, perhaps, from a paper that has never reported that tamoxifen is a known carcinogen.)

The failure of the *Times* to report on the European tamoxifen studies turns out to be entirely consistent with the newspaper's practices, at least as evaluated by Mark Dowie in "What's Wrong with the *New York Times*'s Science Reporting?"—a lead article published in the July 6 edition of *The Nation*. As Dowie concludes in his lengthy review of the publication's science coverage, "In science, even more than foreign or domestic political coverage, the paper tends to side with power—in this case, corporate power. And much of the problem is centered around the work of one very talented and controversial science reporter, Gina Kolata." Dowie's review of Kolata's work is a revealing look at what does—and doesn't—get reported as science news at the *New York Times*. And the losers are readers of the paper who are left with unbalanced reporting on matters of life and death.

Of course, some of us look beyond the daily newspapers to more specialized publications for information on women's health in general and breast cancer in particular. One of the most widely distributed women's health newsletters is the *Harvard Women's Health Watch*. In the June issue, the *Health Watch* published a lead article touting the results of the BCPT-1 as "a landmark in women's health." When BCA's Media Response Task Force objected to the *Health Watch*'s failure to balance its detailed information about the benefits of tamoxifen with similar details about the risks of the drug in healthy women, the *Health Watch* responded with a letter that stated, among other things, that one of the reasons they didn't give statistics on tamoxifen's side effects was that the full set of figures have not yet been released by the NCI.

The absence of complete data from BCPT-1 did not keep the *Health Watch* from trumpeting the trial results in June. And our letters did not keep them from doing so again in July. In another lead article, "Advances in Breast Cancer Research," the July issue discussed tamoxifen and raloxifene as "two promising approaches to prevention." After repeating the "45 percent reduction" figure from BCPT-1, the

Health Watch report on tamoxifen focused on a review in the *Lancet* of a number of studies of tamoxifen. But the *Health Watch* barely noted that the *Lancet* report was about studies of women who had been diagnosed with breast cancer and, therefore, was about secondary not primary prevention. On raloxifene, the *Harvard Women's Health Watch* repeated the interim results of two studies that were presented at the ASCO meeting in Los Angeles and concluded that "Evista can reduce the chance of developing breast cancer, osteoporosis, and possibly heart disease." While promoting both tamoxifen and raloxifene for breast cancer "prevention," the *Health Watch* failed to point out that neither drug has yet been approved by the FDA for use as a preventive in healthy women. (The FDA Oncologic Drug Advisory Committee recommended at its September 2 hearing approval of a new label for tamoxifen that would include prevention. BCA opposes this labeling. For a copy of BCA's written testimony, contact the BCA office.) The pill pushing by the *Health Watch* makes me wonder whether Harvard receives funding from Zeneca (manufacturer of tamoxifen), Eli Lilly, or both.

While the *Harvard Women's Health Watch* is encouraging women to consider tamoxifen and raloxifene for prevention, the NCI is starting a new trial of the two drugs. This trial, officially called BCPT-2, is referred to as the STAR (Study of Tamoxifen and Raloxifene) trial— ironic, since the science seems to be anything but stellar.

Using drugs supplied by the manufacturers, twenty-two thousand women at "high risk" of developing breast cancer will be assigned at random to take either tamoxifen or raloxifene for five years. The biggest problem with the STAR trial is that two unknowns will be tested against each other, with no placebo. This means that since we do not have long-term results from studies of either tamoxifen or raloxifene in healthy women, we won't know what to make of the results. At best, we will learn how the incidence of breast cancer in women on tamoxifen compares with that in women on raloxifene. We will be completely in the dark about how the risks and benefits of either drug compare to taking neither.

Another significant issue is that women who were on the placebo arm of BCPT-1 are being actively recruited for the STAR trial. If enough of them enroll, it will prevent any long-term follow-up for

BCPT-1, because the "control" women whose health histories would be measured against those of women on tamoxifen will also be getting a drug (either tamoxifen or raloxifene), which will make any meaningful comparison impossible. It seems that the NCI is so intent on finding a pill for prevention that it is sacrificing scientific reliability in the process.

As if all of this weren't enough to convince me that someone's off their head, surely the latest from the folks at the City of Hope Cancer Center makes as much sense as the Mad Hatter. Apparently, they have a notion that they can create a nasal spray containing an antihormone to reduce a woman's normal production of progesterone, estrogen, and testosterone. The spray will also contain estradiol and testosterone to replace the "good" hormones that women need for their health. The theory is that removing progesterone and "excess" levels of estrogen will reduce a woman's breast density so that her mammograms will be more readable. The trial is designed for premenopausal women who have a genetic susceptibility to breast cancer or are otherwise at high risk of developing the disease, but the hypothesis on which it is based extends to all women. The sponsor of the study, Balance Pharmaceuticals, Inc., will manufacture and supply the nasal spray.

It seems that some researchers find it easier to "make a better woman" than to design a better detection device or look for the causes of breast cancer as an approach to prevention. Maybe it's time to step back through the looking glass.

October–November 1998

Thinking Out Loud

Toward a New Research Strategy

If you are a regular reader of this newsletter, you won't be surprised to learn that I have many concerns about how—and what—breast cancer research is funded. Fortunately, many activists around the country are thinking about not only what is wrong, but how it might be fixed to get us to the goal of curing and preventing breast cancer. One idea—a call to revamp research into a model similar to the Manhattan Project that generated the atomic bomb for the United States—needs to be explained, discussed, and developed further. And if it withstands careful scrutiny, the idea needs to become a clarion call for change. Where better to begin that process than in the pages of this newsletter?

Breast cancer research is currently carried on by a vast array of both public and private entities. They include pharmaceutical companies, private foundations, research hospitals, academic institutions, and state and federal government agencies. While I can't produce an exhaustive list of even the federal agencies engaged in some form of breast cancer research, off the top of my head I can think of the following: the National Institutes of Health (NIH), National Cancer Institute (NCI), National Institute of Environmental Health Sciences (NIEHS), Centers for Disease Control (CDC: several branches), Environmental Protection Agency (EPA), Office of Women's Health, and the Department of Energy (DOE). And, although I learned at a recent meeting in Washington that there is a "Federal Coordinating Committee on Breast Cancer," I doubt anyone in the federal government or anywhere else would claim with a straight face that we have a co-ordinated strategy for finding a cure for, or understanding the causes of, breast cancer.

The fragmentation throughout the country is even more pro-nounced in the private sector. After all, does the American Cancer Society actually know that the research they are funding is not being replicated by research funded by the Komen Foundation or the Breast Cancer Research Foundation, or being done by Memorial Sloan Ket-tering Cancer Center or anyplace else?

Other aspects of the research process also pose barriers to ac-complishing what can and must be achieved. Research is funded in increments that force scientists to work to renew their grants rath-er than to focus their complete attention on the problem at hand. Uncertainties about what the next "sexy" research area will be keep many outstanding researchers out of the breast cancer field. A desire for academic promotion or personal economic advantage drives far too many researchers either out of breast cancer research or out of research altogether. And many of the pharmaceutical developments related to cancer have been made with public research dollars that are then converted to private profit.

So how do we get to a coordinated research strategy, and how do we implement that strategy in the face of economic pressures that deter us, as a society, from getting where we need to go?

Both strategy and implementation might be achieved with the Manhattan Project model that I mentioned in the opening paragraph of this column. While we need a different name for this idea—"The Rachel Carson Project" comes to mind—the model is based on the no-tion that the same sort of effort that once solved a significant scientific challenge in a short period of time might be used as well for good as it was for harm in the creation of the atomic bomb.

What if we took all the money—public and private—now de-voted to breast cancer research and put it into three or four research centers around the country? The centers would be staffed with the best and brightest scientists now working on issues related to breast cancer treatment and prevention. These scientists would come from a wide range of disciplines and would be guaranteed good salaries and all the research resources they need. They would not have to apply for grants. However, they would be prohibited from using their work to gain academic promotions or from patenting any process or product that resulted from their research. They would be supported until one or more of the centers produced both an effective treatment for breast cancer and an understanding of causes that would permit us to take steps to prevent the disease. A significant financial bonus would be paid to the researchers at the centers that get to the two finish lines first.

Multiple centers would ensure the competitiveness that seems to be necessary to all scientific and medical breakthroughs. The staff of the centers would be selected by a group similar to the Integration Panel of the Department of Defense Breast Cancer Research Program, consisting of breast cancer activists, scientists, policymakers, and industry representatives. This oversight group would be responsible for ongoing review of both the progress and staffing of the centers.

This is just a rough sketch of an idea. If the idea has any merit, a lot of details will have to be worked out. But the first question is whether the idea has validity. So think about it. Talk to your friends about it. Let me know what you think. And if the idea is a good one, BCA, working with other organizations of like mind, will undertake the kind of public education and organizing campaign that can and will end the breast cancer epidemic and put BCA out of business. Because, when all is said and done, that is the goal.

December 1998–January 1999

Rolling the Dice

The headline read "In Breast Cancer Data, Hope, Fear and Confusion." The story by Denise Grady described at length how women overestimate their risk of getting and dying from breast cancer, and the importance of measuring risk over a meaningful period of time like five or ten years. It also pointed out the limitations of the near-legendary statistic that your risk of getting breast cancer is one in eight (*New York Times,* January 26, 1999). Much of the article made sense, but it also made me wonder about what it takes to put numbers about breast cancer in perspective.

Facts are a good place to start. It is true that many people believe that one of every eight women has breast cancer, though the one-in-eight statistic actually reflects an individual's cumulative risk over an eighty-five-year lifetime. It is true that many women fear breast cancer more than they fear heart disease or lung cancer, both of which kill more women. But these misunderstandings have explanations, and those explanations tell us something about where we are in "conquering" breast cancer and in the breast cancer movement.

The one-in-eight statistic is bandied freely about for several reasons. It is a handy shorthand that gives breast cancer advocates a tool to stimulate public clamor for answers to the epidemic. It's an easy number to use to convey a lot of information. As I frequently say in making presentations, the good news is that seven out of eight women will never get breast cancer; the bad news is that thirty years ago the number was nineteen out of twenty. It is also a useful way for public health officials to encourage women to get mammograms. It is almost certainly the case that, by now, at least as far as white middle-

and upper-class women are concerned, both the breast cancer movement and health officials have women's attention.

Increasingly, however, informed medical people, health policymakers, and the media point out that the number overstates a woman's risk of developing breast cancer at any given moment in her life. They say that one of the results of overstating the risk is that women's fear of the disease is out of proportion to their fear of heart disease and lung cancer, both of which are greater threats to women's health.

But I think there is more to it than that. I think women fear breast cancer not because they think their risk is one in eight, but because they have friends and loved ones who have been diagnosed, been treated, and have died of the disease. When I was diagnosed the first time at age forty-one, I was told that only 2 percent of women my age got breast cancer, and I wondered why I seemed to know them all. I think women fear breast cancer because it is about a part of our bodies that makes us female and threatens our sexuality. And I think women fear breast cancer because we perceive that whether we get it and whether we die of it is nothing more than a total crapshoot. It's random, it's deadly, and it goes to the heart of who we are as women. Fear seems to me to be a reasonable reaction.

And that reasonable reaction also explains why women don't fear heart disease and lung cancer as much. We think we can prevent heart disease with diet and exercise. We're confident we can avoid lung cancer by not smoking. And that we're not absolutely right in either case doesn't matter much, because doing these things works for most of us and is good for all of us.

But things aren't so simple in the world of breast cancer. While we hear about exercise reducing breast cancer risk, what gets sold as prevention is and ought to be pretty scary. Whether it's a pill that has numerous side effects, some of which are life-threatening, or prophylactic mastectomies, the choices are simply awful.

So what should we do about how we talk about breast cancer risk? It seems to me that how we talk about it ought to depend on the context in which we are speaking. If we're trying to make a political statement, to get people involved in working to change the research agenda or focus on the precautionary principle, then the one-in-eight number is fine, particularly when put in the context of the one-in-twenty figure of the mid-1960s. If we're trying to explain to a woman what her personal risk is, then it's far more important to talk about how risk changes with age and other factors.

And when we talk about factors that affect breast cancer risk, we need to put those factors in perspective. We know that, taken together, the so-called known risk factors—age, age at menarche, age at menopause, age at first birth, not having children, country of origin, family history of breast cancer, number of breast biopsies and biopsies showing atypical hyperplasia, postmenopausal obesity, and race—account for approximately 30 percent of all breast cancer risk. So to speak of these factors as though they permit us to know what a woman's risk is gives them far more weight than they merit. What happens, for example, if the 70 percent of unknown factors actually, in a given instance, reduce a woman's breast cancer risk? We have to stop treating the part of the picture that we claim to understand as if it were the whole picture.

And we have to stop describing as "risk factors" things that are, in fact, characteristics over which we have absolutely no control. Age, age at menarche, age at menopause, country of origin, family history, results of biopsies, and race are all unchangeable and uncontrollable features of our personal landscapes. Describing these as "risk factors" contributes to the self-blame that has been part of women's experience of breast cancer for far too long.

Finally, we have to keep in mind that all the figures we have about breast cancer risk really tell us nothing about a woman's individualized risk of getting breast cancer because they are based on large population studies, the results of which have no applicability to any particular person. So for any individual woman, at this stage of knowledge, it's almost impossible to know with any certainty what her risk of getting breast cancer is.

Which brings us back to fear. If your future rides on a roll of the dice, you want to know how the dice are loaded. Only public pressure on the research agenda will get us the answers.

April–May 1999

Respecting the Past, Creating the Future

When I was in high school, my best friend in the world was Alma Borenstein. She was smart, fun to be with, and not afraid to take on the difficult issues that confronted those of us who were in our mid- to late teens in the late 1960s. I could talk to Alma about anything and everything, and I did.

College took us in different directions, and we didn't manage to do very well at staying in touch. Nonetheless, I learned from mutual friends that Alma's mother had died of breast cancer while we were in college, and I learned about Alma's own diagnosis when we were both in our thirties.

Alma died of breast cancer ten years ago this spring. Among my peers, she was the first person I knew whose life was cut short by what I now often refer to as "this damned disease." When Alma died, Breast Cancer Action was just getting started, and other than some support groups that were forming around the country and organizations urging women to get mammograms, no one was really talking about breast cancer.

As we celebrate BCA's tenth anniversary year, it's hard to remember that just ten years ago breast cancer was still largely a silent killer and the well-kept secret of hundreds of thousands of women and their families. And while far too little has changed in the diagnosis and treatment of breast cancer, much has changed in the public's awareness of the disease and in people's willingness to discuss their experience with it.

These changes in awareness and public discussion of breast cancer are largely the result of the activities of organizations like Breast

Cancer Action and others that make up the breast cancer movement. Our work is far from finished, but as the young poet Pecolia Manigo says, we've come too far to turn back now. So as we mark BCA's tenth anniversary, I think it is worthwhile to consider what the breast cancer movement might look like ten years from now.

Detection

The next ten years should see substantial progress in the development of more reliable, non-radiation-based technologies for the earlier detection of breast cancer. Breast cancer organizations closely tied to the industries that produce and use mammography equipment will continue to push the outdated technology and to resist changes in public health policy related to breast cancer detection. But more breast cancer organizations will be encouraging the use of these new technologies and free access to them; some organizations will have begun to call for an end to population-based mammography screening, because the data will have strongly suggested that such screening does not reduce breast cancer mortality rates.

Treatment

Progress in the treatment of breast cancer will continue to be slow but real. More treatments that target tumors or cancer cells, rather than all fast-growing cells (including many that are essential to our health), will be available and will be more routinely used in breast cancer treatment. Breast cancer organizations will play an important role in facilitating this progress by having their members serve on peer review for research proposals, bringing to bear a strong voice in support of less toxic, more effective treatments. Breast cancer organizations will also work to ensure that women and men have compassionate access to experimental therapies whenever feasible by pressuring both drug companies and the Food and Drug Administration to make sure that expanded access is an essential element of all Phase III clinical trials.

Treatment Access

Thanks to the efforts of breast cancer activists across the country, every woman screened for breast cancer will have ready access to the best available treatments. In communities everywhere, breast cancer organizations will be involved in efforts to ensure that families whose members are struggling with breast cancer treatment have the practical support they need to get through a difficult time. Alliances between progressive breast cancer organizations and groups working toward universal access to health care will result in significant progress toward ensuring quality health care for all residents of the United States.

Prevention

Despite words of caution from many quarters, including a number of breast cancer organizations, more effort will be devoted to finding pills to "prevent" breast cancer. By the year 2010, we will have begun to see more clearly the adverse consequences of these efforts in the form of health problems in women who have taken the pills as well as in their children. While many breast cancer organizations will continue to place their faith in a pharmaceutical approach to breast cancer prevention, others will have joined Breast Cancer Action in calling for a precautionary public health approach to prevention that focuses on the damage that society is doing to our air, water, and soil. Environmental organizations, health organizations, and these breast cancer organizations will form strong coalitions focusing on the precautionary principle of public health, and public policy will have begun to shift in this direction.

Research Directions

In the next ten years we will begin to learn some of the benefits of unlocking the human genome, and we will also begin to understand the limits of knowing more about human genetic makeup. Research efforts will continue to focus on molecular biology, but the lack of progress in understanding breast cancer, and the continued elusiveness of true cures for the disease, will lead more breast cancer organizations to join Breast Cancer Action in urging new strategies for approaching the breast cancer problem. The Rachel Carson Project—a breast cancer research strategy that takes the potential for profit out of research and frees researchers from the need to constantly seek research grants, while bringing together the best and brightest minds to tackle the problem—will be advocated by a number of breast cancer organizations and will begin to receive serious consideration in research policy circles outside of the National Cancer Institute.

I want people who are now in high school to keep their high school friends into a glorious old age. I believe that over the next ten years the breast cancer movement will have a significant impact on all aspects of breast cancer. And while both a true cure and real prevention will still be in our future in 2010, I believe that—with the continued efforts of BCA and other breast cancer organizations—we will be closer to these goals. Because, as I've heard Pecolia Manigo say, until our dreams are realized, win or lose, still we rise.

July–August 2000

Making Choices

A recent news story described an experiment in which healthy people are being paid by the aerospace company Lockheed Martin to ingest perchlorate, a toxic component of rocket fuel. These folks are being paid $1,000 each so that the company can evaluate whether perchlorate, which has leached into the drinking water in Southern California from a Lockheed jet propulsion plant, is harmful to human health.

The corporation takes the view that the human experiment is acceptable because the U.S. Environmental Protection Agency (EPA) has approved it and because participants are fully informed about the risks and thus are making informed choices. I find this experiment, and the posing of this "choice" to healthy humans, outrageous and unethical.

The Lockheed perchlorate experiment is the latest version of new kinds of "choices" that people are being given involving human experiments and environmental policy. In a thorough and thoughtful report titled "The English Patients: Human Experiments and Pesticide Policy," the Environmental Working Group documents the modern history of human experiments in the development of U.S. policies on pesticides. The report describes the use of these studies by pesticide manufacturers to short-circuit stricter standards for pesticide safety adopted in 1996 and the EPA's failure to follow the ethical rules required for experiments involving humans when formulating pesticide safety standards.

Clearly missing from the EPA-sanctioned experiments is the

premise, inherent in human medical research, that there must be potential benefit from the substance being studied for those who participate in clinical trials. For example, a clinical trial evaluates whether a new drug, either alone or in combination with others, is a better treatment for breast cancer than approved therapies. While the answer from any given cancer clinical trial may be that the new drug is not a better treatment, the trials are undertaken only when evidence points to at least the possibility of benefit.

By contrast, experiments set up to test at what level known toxins are harmful to humans present no possibility of benefit to the trial participants. The best the participants can hope for is that they won't be hurt. But the problem with giving people the "choice" to participate in human experiments with toxic substances extends beyond the lack of any possible benefit. We have been engaged for decades in an uncontrolled human experiment of the effects of a wide range of toxic substances on health and the environment. These substances are released into the environment with little or no consideration for their long-range effects, and people have had and still have no "choice" about exposures to them. Yet manufacturers of some of these substances would now have us accept these exposures based on very small (often fewer than a dozen participants), short-term, unethical experiments.

And who "chooses" to participate in these studies? Who but the most financially desperate among us would voluntarily expose ourselves to known toxins? Under these circumstances, does the concept of "choice" even apply?

The first *Webster's* dictionary definition of the word *choose* reads: "to select, especially freely and after consideration." The dominant culture thus tells us that choice is a good thing, the ultimate expression of freedom. In fact, choices that aren't free have their own name in English—they are called *Hobson's choices*, named for the seventeenth-century stable owner who required every customer to "choose" the horse nearest the door.

This is a brave new world in which the so-called choices presented to the Lockheed trial participants—whether to expose themselves to a known toxin in exchange for money—are vastly different from the world of choices that confronts women and men diagnosed with breast cancer. The choices faced by breast cancer patients—which surgery to have, whether to have a sentinel node biopsy, whether to have chemotherapy and, if so, which chemotherapy to have—are all questions posed as decisions that patients, hopefully in collaboration with their health care providers, must make. And while many people find these choices daunting, most of us have been trained to see choice as positive, even when the things we have to choose among are less than optimal.

Breast Cancer Action has always believed that people are entitled to be fully informed so that they can make the best choices for themselves as they make decisions related to breast cancer diagnosis and treatment. But choices that people with breast cancer are forced to make are between real options that carry potential benefits as well as risks.

Before I was diagnosed with breast cancer, my first strong association with the concept of choice was with the notion that women should be free to choose whether and when to have children. But it was not long before I noticed the concept of choice being turned on its head, framed not as allowing people to make the best decisions for themselves but as assuring that corporations could conduct themselves in any way they wished, so long as people were apparently free to "choose" whether to participate or not.

For example, when it became clear that substances toxic to women's reproductive systems were in use on some industrial production lines, the manufacturers framed the issue as a woman's right to choose what work she did rather than as the producer's responsibility to provide a safe working environment for all of its employees.

In every aspect of our lives as citizens, we should be entitled to make true choices. How can we put a stop to things like the Lockheed human experiment and promote new ways of looking at human health and "choice"?

Maybe the best way to begin to change the world is to change how we talk about things. Bob Erwin, a wonderful breast cancer activist, once passed on to me the following observation:

> If the habit of language changes,
> then the way of thinking changes,

then the perception of need changes,
and someone just might come up with a solution.

In the context of things like the Lockheed experiment and other situations that present no possibility of benefit, maybe we should stop using the word *choice* and instead use words like *greed* or *damage control*.

March–April 2001

Living on the Edge

One of BCA's core principles is the recognition that structural changes in society are needed to accomplish our mission, which is to inspire and compel the changes necessary to end the breast cancer epidemic. At the same time, we serve individuals by advocating for less toxic, more effective treatments that are readily accessible to everyone who needs them.

Because things that help individuals may have adverse consequences in the broader social perspective, BCA often walks a fine line between addressing the needs of individuals and advocating for the broader policy changes that will ultimately permit us to put the organization out of business. A recent news story about a compound that may reduce hair loss during chemotherapy illustrates the challenge we face.

When I underwent six months of chemotherapy treatment in 1993–94, one of the hardest aspects of the treatment was the loss of most of my hair. And while what the public saw—at least when I took off my black Stetson—was the loss of hair on my head, my reality was more intense. Every morning when I looked in the mirror after my shower, I was struck by how my virtually hairless body looked like that of a preadolescent girl. It was a constant and painful visual reminder of how sick and dependent breast cancer and its treatment had made me.

At the time, if someone had asked, I certainly would have said that I would be thrilled by the development of breast cancer treatments that wouldn't cause women to lose their hair. So it was no surprise to me that the press could find women currently in treatment for breast cancer who were delighted by an announcement by Glaxo Wellcome in January: the pharmaceutical company has developed a compound that reduces, by as much as 50 percent, chemotherapy-induced hair loss in up to 70 percent of the rats on which it was tested.

Though the substance has not yet been tested in humans and will require further animal testing before human tests are even considered, the development received extensive press coverage. "Hair loss is one of the most difficult parts of the therapy because it reminds patients every day of what they're going through," said Stephen T. Davis, the author of the study. "This could really have some value for patients." Dr. Davis is certainly right about the value of finding a way to prevent chemotherapy-induced hair loss for chemotherapy patients.

I am now nearly seven years past the end of my chemotherapy treatment, and my experiences as a breast cancer activist and the staff leader of what someone recently called "the thinking person's breast cancer organization" have led me to think about the broader implications of developments like this. While I certainly hope that women and men will soon be able to avoid the devastation of hair loss from chemotherapy treatment, I am concerned about what this development says about the immediate future of breast cancer treatments, what it means about the current direction of cancer research, and what its implications are for society's perception of the cancer epidemic.

What does the nature of this research tell us about the future of treatments for breast and other cancers? Glaxo Wellcome appears to be betting that by the time (some years from now) that this research produces any hair loss benefit for cancer patients, there will be a large enough market to support the expenses associated with it. Does this mean that all of the promised "breakthroughs" in cancer treatment to more targeted, less toxic therapies are much further off than the National Cancer Institute and the biotech industry would have us believe?

It seems to me that the pharmaceutical company's investment is evidence of its belief that, for the foreseeable future, most women diagnosed with breast cancer who undergo chemotherapy treatment will continue to receive highly toxic, systemic treatments that cause hair loss and other considerable harms. The outcome of the NIH's Consensus Conference on Adjuvant Therapy for Breast Cancer confirms my impressions on this score.

The investment of significant resources into the development of a variety of compounds that might reduce or eliminate hair loss from chemotherapy treatment is also evidence that the current direction of most cancer research is on treatment and its side effects, rather than on true cancer prevention. While people and organizations at the grassroots level increasingly demand that attention be focused on why there is so much cancer and what might be done to prevent it, the cancer industry focuses its considerable resources on finding profitable treatments rather than on finding the causes of breast cancer.

The wide and growing gap between what cancer policymakers and researchers are doing and what the public believes they should be doing is highlighted by research like Glaxo Wellcome's. Not surprisingly, the media reports give glowing commendations to the pharmaceutical company's approach and focus on the potential individual benefits of the research rather than on the broad social consequences of the raging cancer epidemic.

This potential treatment for chemo-induced hair loss also has serious implications for what society perceives about the breast cancer epidemic and therefore our ability to galvanize public pressure to end it. When I see a woman in a public place wearing a turban or a scarf wrapped around her evidently bald head, I can be almost certain that she has joined the dreaded sisterhood of the cancer epidemic. The image quickly conveys to me the devastation of breast cancer and its treatments.

From a social perspective, the development of compounds that mask or eliminate the side effects of systemic chemotherapy treatments will make the realities of breast cancer even more invisible than they already are, and it may divert public attention from the urgency of the need for true prevention and less toxic, more effective treatments. But they will not make those realities or needs go away.

In 1980, black lesbian feminist Audre Lorde wrote in her book *The Cancer Journals* about why she refused to wear a prosthesis and the implications of her choice:

Prosthesis offers the empty comfort of "Nobody will know the difference." But it is that very difference which I wish to affirm, because I have lived it, and survived it, and wish to share that strength with other women. If we are to translate the silence surrounding breast cancer into language and action against this scourge, then the first step is that women with mastecto-mies must become visible to each other. For silence and invis-ibility go hand in hand with powerlessness. By accepting the mask of prosthesis, one-breasted women proclaim ourselves as insufficients dependent upon pretense. We reinforce our own isolation and invisibility from each other, as well as the false complacency of a society which would rather not face the results of its own insanities.

By the time Audre Lorde died of breast cancer in 1992 at the age of fifty-eight, the silence around the disease was beginning to break as women with breast cancer began to find each other and speak out in large numbers. Yet our invisibility to much of the rest of world per-sists. By removing from public view the impact of breast cancer and its treatments, we make it easier for people to pretend that society does not have a breast cancer problem, and we make it harder to gal-vanize public pressure to end the epidemic.

So while I hope that individual women will soon have available to them ways to decrease the devastating effects of breast cancer treat-ment, I am concerned that when this happens it will only become more difficult to advance the social policies that would mean that women don't have to face breast cancer treatment at all.

As the executive director of Breast Cancer Action, I know that the organization often lives on the narrow ledge that separates what individuals need and want from what would benefit society as a whole. It's not always a comfortable place to be, but our willingness to be there is one of the things that makes us "the thinking person's breast cancer organization."

May–June 2001

Breast Cancer Treatment

Promise versus Reality

There's an ad I've seen on television recently featuring a relatively young African American woman who says that, while she would certainly never have wanted to get breast cancer, this was a good time for it to happen because there are so many drug treatments available. Thanks to those treatments, the woman says, she is cancer-free. The ad is paid for by a pharmaceutical trade group.

In another ad, cyclist and cancer "survivor" Lance Armstrong touts the day in the near future when his toddler son will have a credit card–sized piece of plastic that carries the details of his genetic make-up, allowing doctors to see and treat cancer long before it becomes a problem.

Hardly a week goes by without an announcement in the press of a promising new treatment for breast cancer, or a feature story about the increasing individualization of breast cancer care made possible by an improved understanding of how breast cancer develops. But for the vast majority of breast cancer patients, the reality is cookie-cutter treatment based on a recipe that is driven entirely by stage of disease: a combination of surgery (slash), radiation (burn), and chemotherapy drugs (poison) that really varies very little from one patient to the next.

I often wonder why the gap between what is promised in the lab (and on TV) and what is delivered in the clinic continues to widen. I suspect that the explanation lies partly in what I think of as the current cancer culture, partly in the economics of cancer, and partly in the increasing dysfunction of the health care system in the United States.

The culture of cancer in twenty-first-century America is one of hope and hype, as the TV ads described above demonstrate. With frequent assertions by the National Cancer Institute, the American Cancer Society, and other members of the cancer establishment that we are "winning the war" on cancer, as well as enthusiastic media reports about promising developments in treating the disease (usually in mice), the public can't help but believe that the big breakthrough in cancer treatment is right around the next corner, if it hasn't arrived already.

Given the hype from the cancer establishment, who can blame people newly diagnosed for expecting that the treatment they will be offered will be far better—less toxic and more effective—than the treatment their mother's generation had? And who can blame those with metastatic disease from believing that the right treatment for them exists, if only they can find it?

The truth is that the vast majority of individuals diagnosed with breast cancer are still offered a combination of surgery, chemotherapy, and radiation that not only is substantially the same from patient to patient but also—except for the extent of the surgery—differs very little from the treatments their mothers would have been offered. And there is still no known treatment that will guarantee a "cure" to people whose breast cancer has metastasized.

The economics of cancer treatment are another part of the story. Though billions of dollars are spent every year in developing new cancer treatments, very few of these treatments ever make it into the clinic. The ones that do have been the subject of such intense effort and investment that for the drug companies to not only recoup their investment but also make a profit, large numbers of people must receive the treatment. It's because so many people get breast cancer that pharmaceutical and biotech companies are targeting the disease. This reality of cancer economics brings to mind the tale of what Willie Sutton is said to have answered when asked why he robbed banks: it's where they keep the money.

For people with breast cancer, this means that while there have been some new therapies introduced into standard breast treatment in recent decades, they have tended to be added to the "standard" treatment rather than given to patients based on the individual characteristics of their disease.

One place where the culture and economics of the disease come together is in the relentless focus on the genetics and molecular biology of breast cancer. These minute aspects of cancer development lead not only to the hope and hype that characterize the culture of cancer, but also to investments (and press releases) by drug companies hoping literally to capitalize on genetic or molecular treatment interventions. While investors and drug companies look for research clues that will bring about continued funding and, ultimately, marketable products, the public is led to believe that each bit of cancer news has true meaning for patients. But the reality is that much of what we understand about genetics and the molecular biology of breast cancer has no real implications for the treatment that patients receive today.

Genetic testing for breast cancer is a good example of this reality. For some years now, we have been able to examine the BRCA-1 and -2 genes for mutations. When I last looked closely at the test, it could find more than four hundred mutations on the BRCA-1 gene alone. The development of the test was announced to great fanfare, and the tests are still heavily marketed to breast cancer patients and patient advocacy organizations. Many breast cancer centers—hospital profit centers built around a highly profitable disease—offer genetic counseling and testing. But what no one can offer is an understanding of the implications of any particular mutation in relation to the development of breast cancer. What we can do in the lab with genetic testing does not translate to anything useful in the clinic.

Similarly, we now have the ability to measure the angiogenesis activity (blood vessel growth) occurring in a particular breast tumor. The ability of a tumor to develop blood vessels is believed to be an indication of the tumor's potential to metastasize. Unfortunately, we don't yet have treatments that can safely inhibit it. So while we can measure more things in relation to breast cancer, we don't have interventions to address what those measurements tell us.

The gap between what is happening in research labs and what is happening to breast cancer patients in the clinic is also the result of the realities of the health care system. A recent story in the *Wall Street*

Journal explained that cost pressures are driving many major cancer centers to discourage people with advanced disease from coming to them for second (or third, or fourth) opinions. Just when people need medical advice the most, the system by which costs are reimbursed by insurance companies and government health plans forces care providers to turn their backs.

People with financial resources, good connections, and the personal wherewithal necessary to locate information about new treatments are still able to get to the doctors they need to see and to get treatments that may help them. For the most part, however, doctors treating cancer have neither the time nor the resources to stay informed about the latest treatments or how to get them, regardless of patients' means and insurance status. As a result, the vast majority of people get a very different kind of care from what we see on the news.

Most people are treated in community or public health hospitals, or through managed care systems that do not encourage or allow doctors to provide cutting-edge care. The result is that most cancer patients get what the health care system offers, and that care is more likely to be one-size-fits-all than individualized. The thousands of cancer patients who either don't have health insurance or lack the personal resources to pursue the care they need may not get even that.

So the next time you hear about a new breast cancer breakthrough, ask what it really means for patients' lives and who has access to it. If the answers are less than meets the eye, send a letter to the editor or call the television station to complain. Until we can narrow the gap between promise and reality of breast cancer treatment, we need to work to change the public's understanding of both.

September–October 2001

Exercise Your Mind

Just about every day, it seems, someone proudly announces to me that she or he has signed up to do some walk, run, or mountain climb to raise money for "the fight against breast cancer." Because these folks know that I'm both a woman living with breast cancer and a breast cancer activist, I think they expect me to be deliriously happy at their effort. But I'm not. These events are merely part of the breast cancer industry's new crusade to get thousands of people to sign up for activities without thinking too much—or at all—about the consequences of what they are doing.

The trend seems to have started with the Susan G. Komen Foundation's Race for the Cure, which was held in ninety-eight cities in 1999.[1] Now it extends to mountain climbs, bike rides, river trips, and walkathons. The objective of these adventures is quite broad: to raise money for breast cancer. I don't know how much money all of these events together raise, and I don't think anyone does. But the amount raised in just one walk is probably a good indicator of how big the money pot is: the Avon Breast Cancer 3-Day walk from Los Angeles to Santa Barbara, California, in 1998 raised $7,793,000.[2] Assuming that the Avon 3-Days subsequently held in other cities raise as much (exact figures were unavailable at press time), multiply that amount by the four cities that became part of the chain in 1999 (with Atlanta, Chicago, and New York), and you start to get the picture. That's over $31 million "for breast cancer" last year alone. And this year the event has expanded further to include Boston, San Francisco, and Washington, D.C.

According to Avon, the cosmetics company that not only sponsors the three-day walks but also heavily markets pink ribbon

merchandise, the proceeds from the walk are awarded to breast cancer organizations that help women who are medically underserved.
That's a laudable purpose, and I'm sure that medically underserved
women can benefit greatly from $31 million. What could be better?

But there is less to this story than meets the eye. In terms of who
participates, how the money is raised, how much is distributed, and
which services are funded, the Avon walks are a striking example of
the way corporations play on legitimate concerns about breast cancer to get people to do things that are far less meaningful than they
appear.

To register for an Avon walk, you have to be at least seventeen
years of age, have health insurance, and agree to raise (or donate)
$1,800 before the walk starts. While Avon also solicits corporate
sponsorships, the vast majority of the funds are raised through individual pledges. In the Los Angeles–Santa Barbara walk, more than
$7 million was raised by the walkers. In exchange, participants get
to walk fifteen to twenty-five miles a day, sleep in tents, and have the
wonderful sense of accomplishing something very difficult with other
people who are equally committed to the cause.

This method of fund-raising—requiring participants in the
event to raise a considerable amount of money—proved successful
with Tanqueray's AIDS Ride and is now used by a number of breast
cancer outdoor adventures. The entry fee and, in the case of the Avon
walks, the health insurance requirement are both powerful barriers
to the participation of any but the most privileged in society. While
poor women might well benefit as much from the physical exercise
and camaraderie that come out of these strenuous physical events, the
entry requirements are prohibitive for them.

There is also the question of how the $7.79 million raised in
the LA walk was distributed. As it turns out, only $5.02 million went
to breast cancer organizations. The rest—36 percent of the money
raised—was spent on what the event producer characterizes as "walker support," administrative (including the producer's fee), and marketing expenses. That means that for every dollar a walker receives
in pledges, less than 65 cents gets anywhere near a breast cancer organization. Whether you are a walker asking for pledges or a person
who has pledged funds to support a walker, wouldn't it make far more

sense to give your dollars directly to the breast cancer organizations you want to support? After all, that way 100 percent of your money would go to a breast cancer cause, instead of 65.

Finally, there's the issue of what programs benefit from the funds that do end up at breast cancer organizations. Avon distributes the net proceeds (the amount left over after the event producer's expenses and fees are paid) to the National Alliance of Breast Cancer Organizations (NABCO). For a fee (a NABCO spokesperson declined to disclose the amount), NABCO redistributes the remaining funds to organizations promoting "breast health" awareness for underserved women. What this amounts to is millions of dollars devoted to encouraging women to do breast self-exams and to get mammograms and clinical breast exams. None of the funds may be used for actual screening; the money can only be used for programs that encourage women to get screening.[3] And not a dime can be used to make sure that these underserved women get treatment if it turns out they have breast cancer. In fact, I'm not aware of any outdoor adventure that raises money to make sure women who have breast cancer get treatment. Nor is any of the funding guaranteed to be paid to organizations in the communities where the walks take place.

A full-page newspaper ad for the Avon 3-Day describes the walk as "the biggest event of its kind ever undertaken in the fight against breast cancer" and "a whole new way to get outdoors and make a difference." And the Avon Web site proclaims that "throughout time people have made great journeys that changed the course of history. Now it's our turn."

Indeed, it is our turn. Make a difference; change the course of history. Think before you agree to do (or sponsor someone for) an outdoor fund-raising adventure. Ask where the money will end up and refuse to support events if you can't get the answer to that question or if the answer you get doesn't suit you. Put your money where your heart is. Then, if you're inclined to walk for the cause, put on your sneakers and head to a local breast cancer organization to volunteer.

Since this article appeared, Avon has made some changes in the way it distributes the funds raised by the walk.

March–April 2000

Notes

1. The first cancer-related fund-raising campaign was also focused on "early detection" education. In 1933, the American Society for the Control of Cancer (later to be renamed the American Cancer Society) launched its Women's Field Army to recruit women to report of periodic physicals that might detect early signs of cancer. The volunteers who made up the Women's Field Army paid an enlistment fee of $1, providing the primary source of funds of the ASCC. See Ellen Leopold, *A Darker Ribbon* (Boston: Beacon Press, 1999), 165–66.

2. See the Pallotta TeamWorks Web site (www.pallottateamworks.com). Pallotta TeamWorks is the creator and producer of the Avon 3-Day walks. Best known for its development and promotion of Tanqueray's AIDS Rides, the firm has come under intense scrutiny from some AIDS activists because of its fund-raising practices and its initial failure to disclose its financial records. See "Open Wide, AIDS Ride," *Poz* (October 1998).

3. The Avon Breast Health Access Fund application is available on the Web at www.nabco.org or through the BCA office.

The Crazy Days of Autumn

Last fall I celebrated my seventh year as the executive director of Breast Cancer Action and my eighth year as a breast cancer activist. I also witnessed the craziest Breast Cancer Awareness Month—what many activists call Breast Cancer Industry Month—I've seen yet. I think, and I certainly hope, that it reflects a growing comprehension of the breast cancer problem and what it will take to end it.

Hardly a day went by during October that didn't present an opportunity to run, walk, or buy something in order to increase breast cancer awareness. But few if any of those activities helped advance a better understanding of what is causing breast cancer, what we can—or can't—do now to truly prevent the disease, how many people are facing breast cancer without access to high-quality health care, or what women and men confront today in terms of treatment options. While more and more companies claimed to care about women by slapping a pink ribbon on a product you could buy, another woman was being diagnosed with breast cancer every two and a half minutes.

This disconnect between all the corporate activity and the harsh realities of the disease prompted Breast Cancer Action to launch our Think Before You Pink® campaign. The premise was that buying a product or doing a walk will not help prevent breast cancer, improve treatment, or guarantee effective care for everyone who needs it. It will take the kind of political work that BCA activists are doing to realize that goal.

The response to the campaign was remarkable. Our quarter-page *New York Times* ad launching the campaign ran in late October, and press interest continued for nearly a month thereafter. As I talked to more and more reporters, it became clear to me that BCA was once again giving voice to a concern that was bubbling just beneath the surface of public awareness. I spoke to so many people who told me that something about all the cause-related marketing for breast cancer—from pink Kitchen Aid mixers to pink ribbons in every store's display window—gave them a yucky feeling that they couldn't quite explain until they read about our campaign.

The reaction to Think Before You Pink® reminded me of something that anthropologists refer to as the "hundredth monkey" phenomenon. The concept comes from the observation that in forests throughout the world, ninety-nine monkeys can be doing something that other monkeys aren't doing and haven't thought of, but when a hundredth monkey does this same thing, all of a sudden all of the monkeys everywhere begin doing it. In other words, when only a limited number of people know of a new way of doing or thinking about something, it may remain the conscious property of only those people. But at some point, when one more person tunes in to that new awareness, a field is strengthened enough for that awareness to be picked up widely.

The resonance created by Think Before You Pink® reached people in ways that surprised even us at BCA. For instance, a producer for a syndicated radio show hosted by conservative commentator Barry Farber contacted me for an interview. Mr. Farber is about as far to the right politically as I am to the left. But our worldviews came together when he saw the *New York Times* ad, and he called me because it so reminded him of the ways in which people are ripped off, day in and day out, by companies that are really only trying to advance their bottom line. My radio interview with Barry Farber was another important reminder that our assumptions about what people will think are often wrong—and that we can always find common ground if we know where to look for it.

Of course, we got lots of hostile responses to Think Before You Pink® as well, many of them from people working for companies that run pink ribbon promotions. The e-mail messages we received from a couple of people at General Mills—the parent company of Yoplait, which brings us the Save Lids to Save Lives breast cancer promotion—were particularly outraged, seemingly out of proportion to the issues we were raising. It prompted us to wonder why.

A little digging into the contents of Yoplait yogurt revealed that General Mills deserves to be on the list of companies that, like BMW and Ford Motor Company, for example, engage in "pinkwashing": branding their products with pink ribbons to cover up the extent to which they contribute to the breast cancer epidemic.

Maybe the reason for General Mills's pinkwashing has to do with how Yoplait is made. Apparently Yoplait is made from dairy products that contain bovine growth hormone (BGH), a substance that has been linked to an increase in breast cancer risk. BCA learned this by contacting the customer service department at the Yoplait division of General Mills, where a spokesperson stated flat-out that "no Yoplait dairy product is BGH-free."

While Think Before You Pink® kept us plenty busy in October and beyond, BCA had many other things to do during Breast Cancer Industry Month. BCA was again involved in organizing the annual Cancer Industry Tour in downtown San Francisco, demonstrating outside the offices of companies and charities that work to keep us from taking a serious look at why so many people in our community are confronting a cancer diagnosis. We also helped to celebrate the selection of Raven~Light, one of the Bay Area's best-known breast cancer activists, as a Lifetime Television "Breast Cancer Hero." And we responded to dozens of press stories on breast cancer issues.

In the midst of all of this activity, we were surprised to get lots of calls and questions about the problem of cancer in Marin County, a region immediately north of San Francisco. We have known for a long time that breast cancer rates—as well as prostate cancer rates—are very high in this county, which is characterized by beautiful rolling hills and a generally well-to-do and well-educated population. Marin's breast cancer rates, which have skyrocketed in the past several years among women forty-five to sixty-five, have been the focus of a great deal of research attention and national press. So why did an organization calling itself the Marin Cancer Project run television ads that asserted—through images of people stepping on or over corpses—that no one was paying attention to the cancer problem in Marin County?

The ads were not only callous but also misleading. They seemed to be an example of how the rich get richer, even when it comes to cancer, while the poor are ignored. Lots of people and organizations are paying attention to the cancer problem in Marin. What we need is the same kind of attention—and resources—devoted to the breast cancer problem in low-income neighborhoods in the Bay Area, such as Bayview–Hunters Point and Richmond, as well as in East Los Angeles, "Cancer Alley" in Louisiana, and other poor neighborhoods throughout the United States.

Reflecting on all that happened in October, I guess it should come as no surprise that the country's leading breast cancer watchdog organization was so busy. But I look forward to a time when, thanks to the hundredth monkey, we don't have to work so hard to convince people that the change we need around breast cancer issues is not the kind you carry around in your pocket.

January 2003

Lessons from Long Island

Results from the long-awaited Long Island Breast Cancer Study were released this summer, and many activists—who have been awaiting the initial findings of the ten-year project—were dismayed.[1] Most reporters, led by *New York Times* science writer Gina Kolata (who has always been skeptical of environmental links to cancer), interpreted the results as proof that pollutants did not cause breast cancer.[2]

But a closer look at the study reveals its limits and points the way to further research that will help us understand why so many of us are getting sick. And taking a step back from the debate that the Long Island study has engendered will help point us toward policies that will alleviate the toxic burden imposed on all of us.

Let's look at the study first. The Long Island Breast Cancer Study was what is known as a "case-control" study of people from two counties on Long Island that appeared to have very high breast cancer rates. The study looked at approximately fifteen hundred women with breast cancer diagnosed between 1996 and 1997 (the cases) and an equal number of women without breast cancer (the controls). Blood samples from each group were examined for evidence of several organochlorine pesticides and PCBs (polychlorinated biphenyl compounds). Other samples were examined for evidence that the DNA had undergone changes from exposure to polycyclic aromatic hydrocarbons (PAHs), a ubiquitous toxin created by cigarette smoke, motor vehicle exhaust, and smoking or burning meat.[3]

Researchers found no association between breast cancer and pesticide exposure or PCBs. They identified a 50 percent elevated risk of breast cancer from PAH exposure, a risk the researchers character-ized as "modest" when compared with, for example, the risk of lung cancer from smoking.

The limitations of this study were identified when the research was first undertaken, and they bear remembering now. The first is the case-control nature of the study. Because breast cancer develops over many years, most researchers believe a case-control study is unlike-ly to reveal how environmental exposures are related to the disease. Instead, a study that follows subjects over a long period of time—a longitudinal study—is much more likely to help us understand the environmental factors contributing to breast cancer. The case-control approach was chosen for Long Island because the activists pushing for this research in the early 1990s wanted answers fast.

While the skyrocketing incidence of breast cancer gives us no reason to be patient, we have learned the hard way that the quick-est research answers are not necessarily the best ones. (Just look at the early studies on hormone replacement therapy and heart disease.) Instead, we need to make the significant commitment of time, ener-gy, and money to longitudinal studies of women and girls, particu-larly those who live in areas with unusually high exposures to toxic substances.

Another major limitation of the Long Island study is that it examined substances—like PCBs and the pesticides dieldrin and chlordane—that have long been banned from production and use in the United States. More than eighty-five thousand chemicals are in daily use in this country, most of which have never been evaluated for their effects on human health. Yet we have good evidence from animal and workplace studies indicating the types of chemicals we should be most concerned about.

But the most challenging limitation of the study, and one shared by almost all environmental health research currently under way, is that scientists have not yet figured out how to measure the combined effects of multiple, long-term exposures to environmental toxins. Af-ter all, no one who lives in an industrialized society is exposed to only one pollutant at a time. Yet that is essentially what the Long Island study looked at. So the strongest conclusion we can draw from the pesticide and PCB information from Long Island is that, by themselves, these things do not appear to be increasing the risk of breast cancer. But we're all exposed to many pollutants, all the time.

Research to illuminate the environmental causes of breast cancer in the world around us and beyond will be expensive and time consuming, and it will require a commitment from activists, scientists, and policymakers. And while this research is under way, we need to let people know what we know and what they can do about it. Rather than minimize the PAH effect as "modest," we ought to be educating the public about ways to control their exposure to PAHs and about the essential political work needed to reduce everyone's exposure to these kinds of substances.

That means working for the widespread implementation of what policy activists refer to as the precautionary principle of public health, or "better safe than sorry." That work must move forward because it will be a long time, if ever, before science can give us the answers we need and are rightly demanding. For while contemporary Western culture has made scientific proof our holy grail, we need to begin to understand that science, like everything else, has limits. In fact, the very process of science—develop a hypothesis, test the hypothesis, and from the results of that test, develop the next hypothesis and test it—is not designed to get us the kinds of answers and "proof" that the public so desperately wants and that the industry continues to tell us has not been achieved.

So as we use the lessons of Long Island to push for better environmental research, we need to realize that reliable answers that develop through that research, if they come at all, will be many years in arriving. We cannot let the process of science hold us back from working now toward policies that will reduce the chemical exposures that we all experience, all the time.

When I was diagnosed with breast cancer at the age of forty-one nearly ten years ago, I quickly learned that what happens to me is out of my hands. I'm one of the lucky ones; I'm still here. But the fate of those who follow rests very much in our hands. We don't have time to despair. There's work to do. We cannot, and will not, give up. Our daughters' and granddaughters' lives are at stake.

November–December 2002

Notes

1. Dan Fagin, "Tattered Hopes," *Newsday,* July 28–30, 2002 (three-part series).

2. Gina Kolata, "Breast Cancer on Long Island: No Epidemic Despite the Clamor for Action," *New York Times,* August 29, 2002.

3. "The Environmental Connection: Recent Research Findings," *BCA Newsletter* no. 62 (November– December 2000).

Waging War, Making Connections

A dear friend and colleague of mine in the cancer movement tells me that you can reframe most issues through a cancer lens. I've been reminded of this often as I think about what our "War on Cancer" and the current U.S. approach to foreign policy have in common.

In both cancer and foreign policy, the U.S. strategy is to advocate and use the most aggressive approaches possible to address a problem. If one chemotherapy drug works well, wouldn't two or a stronger one work better? If supporting opposition forces in Iraq might work to rid the world of a problem like Saddam Hussein, won't all-out war be even better?

In both cancer and foreign policy, we never think seriously about the long-term consequences of the interventions we pursue, since short-term results are the only ones we seem to care about. The result is that we expose individuals (in the cancer realm) and whole societies (in the foreign policy arena) to interventions that may result in serious adverse effects over the long term, but we rarely stick around long enough to find out what those consequences will be. It's not really surprising that we don't know the long-term consequences of giving powerful chemotherapy drugs to younger and younger women with breast cancer when you consider that we have no idea what will happen to the Iraqi children exposed to depleted uranium from U.S. armaments.

In both cancer and foreign policy, we refuse to examine root causes, so that preventing cancer or keeping the international situation from developing into a crisis is impossible. In cancer, when we demand prevention, we are offered powerful pills, the long-term consequences of which are unknown. In foreign policy, when we call for an examination of the behavior that might have led to the terrorist attack on the World Trade Center, we're told that even posing the question is unpatriotic.

In both cancer and current U.S. foreign policy, big business is the driving force, so that news about developments in cancer treatments and advances in American interests abroad are both more likely to be found on the business page than in any other part of the newspaper.

These parallels are important because they help me reframe how I think about connections in the world. One of things distinguishing BCA from a number of other cancer organizations—and one of the reasons I work here instead of elsewhere—is that BCA looks at the cultural, social, political, and economic context in which breast cancer arises and challenges the premises that keep us from seeing clearly what needs to happen to end this scourge.

By framing things in this context, we help to reframe the conversation about breast cancer. We don't need more war analogies about cancer. Let's talk about breast cancer as a human problem instead and start thinking about the human impacts of how we approach the disease.

September–October 2003

※

Solving the Breast Cancer Puzzle

Advancing the Research Revolution

Allow me a ramble here. I promise there's a point to all of what I'm about to say.

Those of you who read *Fortune* magazine will have already seen, and presumably devoured, the cover story from the March 22 issue, tantalizingly titled "Why We're Losing the War on Cancer (and How to Win It)." A BCA member alerted me to the article, and when I read the first half, I was amazed and thrilled that a major mainstream publication had published such an excellent critique of how we fund and do cancer research in the United States. That was the "why we're losing the war" part. The second half of the article—on how to win the "war"— fails unfortunately to come to grips with the critique of the first half. Nevertheless, the article, by Hodgkin's disease survivor Clifton Leaf, provides an excellent framework for thinking about how to change the course of the breast cancer epidemic.

Of course, we at BCA have been thinking, writing, talking, and advocating for changes in how we approach research for some time. When we first framed a possible solution, we even gave a name to the idea: the Rachel Carson Project. Over time, we've talked to lots of people about the problem(s): the lack of coordination of breast cancer research, the traditional "hypothesis-driven" basic science approach, and the piecemeal funding mechanisms, to name a few. We broadly described a model to solve these problems—one that funds multidisciplinary, centrally and adequately funded competitive research centers focused on finding answers to particular questions. We call this "outcome-driven" research. And BCA activists have urged the California Breast Cancer Research Program to serve as the testing ground for the model.

At the San Antonio Breast Cancer Symposium last December, it finally dawned on me that a good analogy for the problems we have in solving the central issues in breast cancer is that of a puzzle. Breast cancer is a puzzle, and the time, energy, and billions and billions of dollars that have been spent trying to solve the puzzle have given us lots of pieces that will be central to understanding and solving it. But there are no puzzle masters who are bringing those pieces together into a recognizable framework. Plus, the National Cancer Institute/American Cancer Society culture of scientific research is a significant barrier to achieving what we need to achieve.

The crackerjack BCA staff has been thinking hard about these issues, soliciting the input of concerned activists and researchers. We've come up with a new name for our project, the Breast Cancer Puzzle Project: Reclaiming the Research Agenda. And we've identified what we see as the four central issues that need to be resolved if we're ever going to put BCA out of business. They are:

- Who needs treatment and who doesn't: which "breast cancers" will never become life-threatening?

- How can we more effectively and less toxically treat metastatic disease, or prevent aggressive breast cancers from becoming metastatic?

- What scientific tools can be developed that will help us make the link between information about environmental exposures (body-burden data) and health-outcome data?

- Why do different racial and ethnic groups have different breast cancer incidence and mortality rates, and what can be done to successfully address those differences?

To get the answers to these questions, we need to start demanding that scientists address them. And we need to start funding the scientists willing to devote their attention to them.

Pie in the sky? Not really. There are folks willing to rethink how we do research, many of them at the California Breast Cancer Research Program (CBCRP). After a three-year priority-setting review, this program is trying to break the mold, preparing to venture into outcome-driven research.

As a former member of the California Breast Cancer Research Council, the program's advisory committee, I had the honor of being invited to the recent meeting where research priorities were set for the next three to five years. It was clear to me as I participated in the meeting (up until the time for voting, a privilege reserved for current council members) that the council members and program staff were being extremely thoughtful about the program's mission to reduce the burden of breast cancer on California without duplicating what other research programs are doing.

The council made the decision to take a significant step back from funding what it has been funding for the past ten years and to refocus its efforts. The CBCRP is now prepared to devote 30 percent of its funds over the next five years (a total conservatively estimated at $17.25 million) to outcome-driven research, which it has dubbed "Program Initiatives." The council will attempt to develop two such initiatives: one on the environmental and lifestyle causes of breast cancer; and one on the racial, ethnic, and social disparities in the burden of breast cancer.

Over the next several years, the CBCRP will use its resources to try to figure out the best way to do this outcome-driven work. The current plan is to set up one or more task forces to look into the feasibility of approaching key questions on these two topics. As with all CBCRP efforts, both breast cancer scientists and activists will be involved in the task force, as will policymakers, scientists, and advocates from other fields.

BCA will be invited to participate on this task force, and we will work closely with CBCRP over the next few years to help shape this groundbreaking effort. It will be a great opportunity for BCA activists who want to be involved in restructuring research.

So, pie in the sky? Maybe. But we're getting closer to the sky all the time. California is once again leading the way. Keep in mind that from the beginning of the breast cancer movement, activists have been the moving force behind every change in this field. The Breast Cancer Puzzle Project is an idea whose time has come—because you demanded it.

March 2004

Forests and Trees

Reflections on Pink Bracelets and Narrow Visions

You haven't been out much lately if you haven't seen yellow wrist-bands around. Promoted by and benefiting the Lance Armstrong Foundation, they were inspired by the cyclist's amazing story as both a cancer survivor and the record-holding winner of the Tour de France, the most grueling of all bike races. The foundation says that "yellow is the color of hope, courage, inspiration, and perseverance." It also happens to be the color of the shirt worn by the winner of the Tour de France.

You probably won't be surprised that I'm not wearing one of these bracelets. But when they first appeared, it struck me that they give visual evidence of the number of people—now more than ten million—who are living with a cancer diagnosis in this country alone. In marked contrast to things like the American Cancer Society's Look Good, Feel Better program, which while helping women in treatment also helps mask the human and social impact of cancer, these little yellow bands are easily identified. What if all or most of us who have had cancer wore them? Wouldn't the world start to literally see the scope of the cancer epidemic?

Not surprisingly, the wristbands are being worn not only by folks who have had cancer but also by those inspired by Armstrong's remarkable story. So what I hoped for is not going to happen. But now we're seeing pink wristbands signifying—you guessed it—breast cancer. Susan Love is raising funds with one; Target is selling pink "Share Beauty, Spread Hope" bands benefiting the Breast Cancer Research Foundation; and the Susan G. Komen Breast Cancer

Foundation offers its own "Sharing the Promise" pink wristbands. I'm sure that many other organizations will be in on the act soon. And, from where I sit, this will only make matters worse.

I'm not going to go off on my anti-pink rant; you can read plenty about that elsewhere. What I am concerned about is that, one more time, the breast cancer movement is separating itself from the rest of the cancer world in ways that I'm afraid will only add to a growing sense—and frustration—among many that breast cancer gets attention out of proportion to other cancers, and that breast cancer advocates don't see themselves as part of a larger cancer community. For once, can't breast cancer people be one of the many trees in the forest of folks living with cancer?

I know this must sound strange coming from someone who works at Breast Cancer Action. But many of the issues we deal with are issues for all kinds of cancer. And BCA has for years framed its work as a wedge: since women are more concerned about breast cancer than any other disease, we address things through the lens of breast cancer in a way that helps people understand that if we change what is happening in breast cancer, we change all of women's and men's health.

There are certainly times when the issues we confront in breast cancer are unique to the disease. But I think we do everyone a great disservice when we separate ourselves in unnecessary ways. Would there be some harm in women who care about breast cancer wearing a yellow wristband? Is there anything to be gained by separating ourselves with pink ones? Can't we sometimes work with a bigger vision that sees what we have in common, instead of what separates us?

And speaking of narrow visions, a prize on this score goes to some of the folks involved with the National Breast Cancer Coalition (NBCC) who are upset that BCA's Breast Cancer Puzzle Project includes the Department of Defense (DoD) Breast Cancer Research Program among the many institutions being asked to work together to solve the breast cancer puzzle. NBCC has long thought of the DoD program as its wholly owned subsidiary, so it's not surprising that NBCC advocates feel protective of the program. But the DoD is one of many, many breast cancer funding agencies, and it, like the others, needs to be held accountable to a wider public. It's just one tree in the research funding forest.

March–April 2005

Fifteen Years of Activism

Standing on Many Shoulders

BCA is celebrating fifteen years of activism this year. When September rolls around, I will mark ten years as executive director of this wonderful organization. Many people who know me and Breast Cancer Action are surprised to learn that the organization existed before I became involved. But the fact is that I am just the person who currently has the privilege of being the public voice for thousands upon thousands of women and men whose voices BCA carries.

Others have had this privilege before me. Some of their names are well known in the breast cancer world: Elenore Pred, Belle Shayer, Susan Claymon, Linda Reyes, Nancy Evans. But it's the many others whose names are less well known, or not known at all, that make what I do, and what each of the previous BCA leaders has done, possible.

In preparing for BCA's fifteenth-anniversary celebration, and thinking about my ten years at the helm, I'm taking time to reflect on all the women and men whose efforts have helped make this organization such a powerful center of the progressive breast cancer movement. Some of them I have never met. Others I knew and worked with, but they have since moved on or, tragically, died. Some of them have spent much of their free time helping others with breast cancer, or confronting the political, economic, and social forces that stand in the way of ending the breast cancer epidemic. Others write an occasional letter to the editor or staff a BCA table at a public event. Some have served on the BCA board of directors; others have worked as

BCA staff or consultants; still others stuff envelopes at the BCA office when they have time.

Some of these people have inspired transformative events at BCA. Linda Reyes, who died in 1994, oversaw the publication of BCA's very first newsletters. Lauren Langford, who died in 1996, helped create BCA's first Web site. Diane Simpson Tompkins directed the first professional membership survey BCA conducted. Collette Sell and Madeleine Ballard managed our first-ever town meeting for breast cancer activists. Carmen Ortiz helped create our Spanish-language newsletter, *Saber Es Poder*. Kendra Klein created the organization's e-alert.

Other people participate in ways that make it possible for BCA to function day in and day out by providing information to people who need it, organizing folks to do something besides worry, pushing policymakers to do the right thing for women with and at risk for breast cancer, or contributing the money that keeps the doors open. No matter how much time or money they give, all of these people make BCA possible.

As I think about all these people, I'm reminded once again that no one who leads an organization does so alone. Like everyone else who works at or with BCA, I walk on paths that have been blazed by the people who led the way before me. In the words of Audre Lorde from her book *The Cancer Journals*, those pathways give us "what [we] need to express the power of [our] knowledge and experience, and through that expression, to develop strengths that challenge those structures within our lives that support the Cancer Establishment."

Lorde also wrote in *The Cancer Journals* about "the mistaken belief that women are too weak to deal directly and courageously with the realities of our lives." The vitality of Breast Cancer Action as it celebrates fifteen years of activism is a testament to just how mistaken that belief is. As John Edwards told his constituency recently in an e-mail to hundreds of thousands of people, the work of Breast Cancer Action provides hope to people living with breast cancer. Audre Lorde saw hope as "a living state that propels us, open eyed and fearful, into all the battles of our lives. And some of those battles we do not win. But some of them we do."

While BCA has lost some battles over the past fifteen years, we are proud of our many victories. By acknowledging and honoring the many hearts, hands, and minds that have brought us to where we are today, we find the strength and energy to continue BCA's work as long as necessary to end this epidemic.

June 2005

Era of Hope, Hype, or Hoax

Is It Time for Change in the DoD Breast Cancer Research Program?

The U.S. Department of Defense (DoD) Breast Cancer Research Program has begun to jump-start progress toward "eradicating breast cancer" and, from the start, it has been strongly influenced by breast cancer advocates—called "consumers" by the DoD. The National Breast Cancer Coalition (NBCC) has played a leading role by training advocates in science, enlisting those advocates in peer review for the program, and selecting the advocates and researchers who serve on the DoD Integration Panel, which sets program priorities for research funding. The laudable goal was to liberate science from the constraints of the traditional NIH (National Institutes of Health) funding model and embolden researchers to work with women living with breast cancer to blaze new and more productive paths leading to better treatments and breast cancer prevention.

Having served as a DoD peer reviewer in the mid-1990s, I am invited to the meetings, called Era of Hope, at which the program reports on its progress.

Over the years I've heard the objectives of the DoD program described in various ways. While the overall vision is "to eradicate breast cancer," the objectives of the program, as described at the 2002 Era of Hope meeting, were to fund research that would translate promising information from the bench to the bedside. In this year's opening remarks Fran Visco, president of NBCC, said that the program's purpose was to find and fund research in the areas where there are gaps in our knowledge about breast cancer.

With more than $1.6 billion and twelve years invested in breast cancer research with DoD's innovative model, it seemed reasonable to expect that reports at the Era of Hope meeting would reveal significant advances, at least toward treating breast cancer more effectively and less toxically. There was certainly a lot of information on the agenda. The abstract book containing brief summaries of the scientific presentations and poster sessions was 538 pages long. Most of the meeting, which covered more than three days, ran nonstop from 7 a.m. until 8:30 p.m.

Yet we heard very little in all of the sessions about anything that is helping patients cope better with a diagnosis today, or preventing the development of breast cancer in women tomorrow. NBCC's e-mailed report on the wonders of the meeting belies the fact that the research funded by the DoD program has yet to result in significant clinical improvement for breast cancer patients. There was a lot of talk about Herceptin at this meeting, building on the excitement arising from the American Society of Clinical Oncology (ASCO) meeting in May.

Some of the advocates at the Era of Hope meeting urged patience. After all, they say, science is a slow process, and progress never comes quickly.

But I see no reason to be patient, as the incidence of breast cancer continues to skyrocket, and we go to more and more funerals. And I wonder whether part of the reason that we haven't seen more progress is that the DoD program, for all its "consumer" involvement, has come to resemble in many ways the research programs it was intended to reinvent. Might some different points of view help redirect this program and get us to answers more quickly?

The intent of Era of Hope, as described in the 150-page program book, was in part "to provide a forum for scientists, clinicians, and breast cancer survivors to share their ideas and to reflect on promising, innovative avenues of research for upcoming years." Yet I was struck, as were others with whom I spoke, by the lack of opportunity during the conference to actually talk with others who attended. Networking opportunities were not part of the agenda. There was no place or time in the meeting plan for advocates to come together to discuss what they were learning or what they thought about the program. There were no opportunities to either ask questions of scientists who presented at plenary sessions or to have in-depth discussions with researchers.

A consumer lounge was created to facilitate interaction between and among "consumers." But the lounge was located in a remote corner of the building and time to "lounge" was a luxury not afforded by the agenda.

Frustrated by the lack of opportunity to connect with other activists and by the lack of useful results from the DoD program, several of us decided to do what activists do—we called a meeting. In a handwritten note that we posted on the meeting message board, we urged advocates who wanted to talk to each other about what was happening at the conference to gather for lunch one afternoon. About forty people showed up, including the public affairs specialist and the consumer liaison for the DoD program.

Our attempts to generate a frank discussion about the conference and the program were somewhat hampered by two advocates who work closely with the DoD program. But a number of good ideas came out of the discussion, some related to the future of Era of Hope meetings and others related to the DoD program in general:

- Create time in the Era of Hope meeting agenda for networking

- Hold a meeting orientation for advocates prior to the event

- Hold a meeting orientation for scientists about working with advocates and the role of advocates in the program

- Allow opportunities during plenary presentations for questions from the floor

- Create an advocate room near the center of meeting activities (things that might happen there include an advocates meeting and a sign-in sheet for advocates to provide contact information for future networking)

- Require presenters to communicate what their work means today for patients or women at risk

- Provide mentors for advocates who want help with science during the meeting
- Plan meal times around opportunities for scientists and advocates to interact
- Open up the Integration Panel to advocates with diverse organizational affiliations and health care professionals who have a working knowledge of less familiar areas, such as integrative medicine (e.g., acupuncture)
- Create a more effective mechanism to ensure funding for promising preliminary research

Our gathering clearly made some of the DoD personnel nervous, but it shouldn't have, particularly given the keynote presentation by Rosabeth Kanter, a Harvard Business School professor whose field of expertise is leadership for change. In articulating the skills needed for innovation, Professor Kanter mentioned several that bear remembering, including keeping an open mind to a wide variety of information and being open to criticism, kaleidoscope thinking (being aware that there can be other approaches), and sharing credit and recognition.

August–September 2005

Meaningful Results

Getting What We Need from Science

I hadn't been back from sabbatical for more than a week when the Sunday night ABC evening news show teased a Monday story about the latest breast cancer breakthrough: a new pill to "prevent" breast cancer. While it took me a few minutes (since my mind was still on something of a breast cancer vacation), I quickly realized that the results must have been from the STAR trial, the study of tamoxifen and raloxifene in healthy women to reduce their risk of breast cancer. When the teaser closed with "Every family that cares about breast cancer will want to see this important story," I braced myself for endless hype.

When I saw the next day's news coverage of the study, I knew that my expectations about hype had been met and even exceeded. But what concerned me more was the failure to provide meaningful information for women with and at risk for breast cancer.

What Matters: Absolute versus Relative Risk

One of the major problems with the way that scientific studies are reported is that in most cases the figures provided represent the relative benefits of the intervention being studied instead of the absolute benefits that an individual woman might experience. In the STAR trial results, which were so widely reported in April, both the National Cancer Institute and the news media (with a few notable exceptions) told us that both tamoxifen and raloxifene reduced breast cancer risk by 50 percent. That's the relative benefit: the percentage you get when you look at the number of women who got breast cancer while on either tamoxifen or raloxifene, compared to the number you would expect to get without the drug, based on the risk of breast cancer in each group.

Women in this trial had an average 3.5 percent chance of developing breast cancer in the next five years. So the 50 percent reduction means, for the individual with this level of risk trying to evaluate whether to take the drug, that her risk would be reduced to 1.7 percent.

Compounding the problem of reporting relative risk information for benefits of drugs is the practice—seen far too often—of reporting the benefits in relative terms but the risks in absolute terms. Since absolute numbers are always smaller than relative ones, this type of reporting leads people to believe that the benefits are always greater than the risks.

Most of the oncology community understands the difference between relative and absolute risk, as does the National Cancer Institute (NCI) and the National Surgical Adjuvant Breast and Bowel Project (NSABP), which runs most of the NCI's major breast cancer trials, including the STAR trial. The NCI and NSABP were intensely criticized in 1998 for touting the relative benefits of tamoxifen for healthy women instead of focusing on the absolute numbers so that healthy individuals could make truly informed decisions about taking the drug. Since then, many articles—both scientific and nonscientific— have been published about the fact that the relevant information for someone trying to decide whether to undergo a particular medical treatment is the absolute risk and benefit information, not the relative information.

It's not hard to understand why drug manufacturers report results in relative terms. After all, what sells drugs better than success? And what looks more like success than relative risk numbers? But it has become tragically clear that the NCI's and NSABP's insistence on touting relative instead of absolute risk information is a result of an increased reliance on "public/private partnerships" that are of greater benefit to private corporate interests than to the general public. It's a scandal that the public needs to look to nonprofit organizations like

BCA for meaningful information about breast cancer treatments. And only public pressure on government institutions like the NCI will end that scandal.

Who Needs What Treatment?

Anyone who has ever been diagnosed with breast cancer quickly confronts the critical question of whether they need treatment beyond surgery. One of the most frequent questions we get at BCA is whether someone diagnosed with breast cancer needs to have chemotherapy.

Patients would not need to ask this question if medical science could tell at the time of diagnosis whether their breast cancer will metastasize (spread to life-sustaining organs) or not. After all, if you knew that your breast cancer would never threaten your life, you would almost certainly skip the experience of chemotherapy and/or hormonal treatments, as well as radiation treatment, since all of these treatments have risks that no one would voluntarily undergo if they could avoid them.

Tragically, despite billions of dollars invested and many decades of research, this information remains unavailable. The good news is that some researchers are actually starting to look for an answer.

A recent retrospective study published in the *Journal of the American Medical Association* indicates that women whose breast cancer is not sensitive to estrogen (ER-negative) may benefit from chemotherapy, but that chemotherapy adds little benefit over hormonal treatments to most ER-positive patients.

Because the study is retrospective, rather than a prospective, randomized clinical trial, and because it shows that some ER-positive patients benefited from chemotherapy in addition to hormonal treatments, we cannot confidently tell any individual with ER-positive breast cancer that she will not gain any benefit from chemotherapy.

In response to the study, researchers have announced the beginning of a ten-year randomized, prospective clinical trial to try to answer this question. Unfortunately for the more than two million women who will be diagnosed with breast cancer in the next ten years in the United States alone, the study's results will not yet be available.

A number of people are wondering why it's taken so long for

the medical research community to focus on the critically important question of who needs what treatment. Breast Cancer Action is determined to continue to push for the answer to this and other unanswered questions regarding breast cancer. This fall, as our contribution to Breast Cancer Industry Month, we will focus the public's attention on the need to figure out whose breast cancer will metastasize.

August–September 2006

BCA's Survey on Aromatase Inhibitors

Meeting the Needs of Patients

I was at the San Antonio Breast Cancer Symposium in 2001 when the first results of a trial looking at an aromatase inhibitor (AI)— the ATAC trial (Arimidex, Tamoxifen Alone, or in Combination)— were presented. I knew from the buzz at the meeting that these results would change practice overnight and that, by the following week, postmenopausal women with breast cancer would be encouraged to take an AI instead of tamoxifen.

I knew a few other things as well from BCA's work, particularly based on what the organization had heard from women when tamoxifen was the treatment of choice. Again, women would want—and need—to know the short- and long-term side effects of this new class of drugs. They would want to know how long the drugs should be taken. They would want to know whether symptoms they were experiencing were truly side effects of the drugs.

Because Arimidex was approved by the Federal Drug Administration (FDA) under its fast-track approval system, the kind of information that women need is not available. FDA rules require drug companies that make products approved under the fast track system to continue to monitor the drug effects once the drug is on the market. But the fact is that very few of these "post-market" trials are actually completed. One reason is the lack of FDA resources. Another is that the pharmaceutical industry is usually more interested in getting drugs to market than in having a complete side effect picture to present.

In late 2002, drug maker AstraZeneca received FDA approval

to market Arimidex as adjuvant therapy for estrogen-receptor or progesterone-receptor-positive breast cancer in postmenopausal women. Very soon thereafter, BCA started hearing from women (whose doctors were recommending the drug) who wanted to know both the side effects of the drugs and how long they should stay on them.

Knowing that the FDA couldn't, and the drug industry wouldn't, collect this information, we decided to do it ourselves. Having been an informal repository for side-effect information of tamoxifen, BCA decided to systematically ask women about their experiences on Arimidex and the two other AIs, letrozole (Femara) and exemestane (Aromasin). After all, patients almost always know before the medical community what side effects they are experiencing as a result of the drugs they are taking. If, in the case of AIs, we could get them to tell us, we could use the power of BCA to communicate that information to women, their doctors, the FDA, and the pharmaceutical industry.

With the help of wonderful volunteers like Diane Tompkins, who helped us design our survey, and Marilyn Zivian, who analyzed the data, BCA staff—headed by our program manager, Brenda Salgado—created the survey, reached out to other advocacy organizations to encourage participation in the survey, and quickly collected a lot of responses.

With this issue of the *BCA Source*, we report on the preliminary results from our AI survey. We will continue to collect, analyze, and release data from the survey so that women one day will know all of the short- and long-term side effects of these treatments, and doctors will know how best to prescribe these drugs.

Information allows people to make informed choices about their care. In the current environment, nonprofit organizations like BCA take on the responsibility to provide this information when government agencies and drug companies don't. While we do that work, we also push for the day when, in the interest of patients and those who care for them, both federal agencies and the pharmaceutical industry provide complete drug information before extensive marketing occurs.

December 2006

Moving beyond the Personal in Environmental Health

M any people are rightfully concerned about their personal exposure to environmental contaminants. At every BCA presentation on breast cancer and the environment, folks ask us what they can
do to reduce incidences of exposures in their daily lives. Though we
do our best to answer these questions, we also know that individual
actions, no matter how well intended, will not be enough to clean
up the toxic mess that we as a society have made. So in addition to
urging people to protect themselves and their families from environmental toxins, we also encourage people to think about how they can
get involved in doing things that will help make personal protections
unnecessary.

The best example of why this matters is one I heard some years
ago from Sandra Steingraber, biologist, poet, and environmental
health activist, when she and I presented together at a conference.
Some people in the audience asked whether Sandra would advise using a filter on showerheads to reduce exposure to the chlorine in water.
Sandra noted that people are exposed to more chlorine through their
skin when they shower than when they drink tap water, so filtering
chlorine out of shower and bath water is a good idea on an individual
basis. But she also noted that when the filters outlive their usefulness,
they have to be disposed of in landfills. Eventually, the chlorine from
the filters will end up back in the environment. Wouldn't it be more
effective to organize the community to demand a water filtration system that is not based on chlorine?

Individual solutions aren't bad, but they rarely lead to the kind of fundamental social changes that are necessary to build a sustainable, relatively toxin-free environment for *everyone*.

Individuals still need to protect their health, but there is rarely a situation in which the only options available are those that stop at the threshold of their homes. For example, if you've decided that you shouldn't use pesticides in or around your home, you can also help educate others about the importance of the choice you are making. If you've chosen to use only body care products that do not have parabens or phthalates in them, you can get involved in the Campaign for Safe Cosmetics to encourage cosmetics companies to make safer products for everyone. If you've decided to use public transit when possible, you can also push car manufacturers to make vehicles that don't depend on fossil fuels, which create exhaust that causes breast cancer and other illnesses.

Much of contemporary American society is focused on individual choice and personal activity, with little regard for the impact of that activity on the common good. Environmental health is one arena where it is clear that only by moving beyond the personal will we ever generate the political will necessary to make the world a better place for everyone. So, the next time you do something to protect your and your family's health, consider how you can take that effort a step further by getting involved with folks who, just like you, want to reverse the tide of toxic exposures.

September–October 2007

Putting Patients First

The Need for Better Standards at the FDA

I have written frequently about the Food and Drug Administration for this column. It has never seemed more important than now to spell out in the clearest possible terms what breast cancer patients need from the FDA and why.

The FDA's recent approval of Avastin (bevacizumab) is the latest case in point. In an open letter to the FDA, we pointed out that with this decision the agency has lowered the bar on the approval of cancer drugs.

Every day seems to bring a new story either about the dangers of drugs long ago approved by the agency or about the undue influence of the pharmaceutical/biotech industry on FDA decisions. As the only national breast cancer organization that has declared its complete independence from funding by pharmaceutical companies (see BCA's Corporate Contributions Policy), BCA is in a unique position to articulate a clear standard for approval of new breast cancer drugs.

In addition, as a result of our in-depth strategic planning process, we at BCA have decided to increase our FDA advocacy efforts, so it is critically important that we be clear for ourselves and for our constituents about how we see the drug approval situation and how we would like to transform it.

There are many drugs approved for breast cancer. (For a list of breast cancer treatment drugs available free or at discounted rates, see our guide to patient assistance programs.) We at BCA believe that any new drug approved for the treatment of breast cancer must be demonstrated to be able to do at least one of the following three things:

- Extend the life of the patient, i.e., improve overall survival (OS)
- Improve the patient's quality of life
- Cost less than therapies already available

Improve Overall Survival

Robert Erwin's article in this issue puts in context how the FDA's recent approval of Avastin for breast cancer treatment came about and why the ruling was so controversial. The debate over Avastin centers on whether the drug's ability to improve progression-free survival (PFS) for some patients should justify its approval for the treatment of metastatic breast cancer patients. While PFS is used increasingly in the cancer field as a surrogate for overall survival, this substitute standard is only useful if, in fact, the surrogate standard can be shown to correlate with what it is meant to stand for: overall survival. In the case of Avastin, as presented to the FDA in December, PFS improved but OS did not. So, consistent with the standard enumerated above, BCA opposed approval of Avastin for breast cancer at the time and was gravely disappointed that the FDA commissioner ignored the recommendation of his committee and granted Genentech's application.

Improve Quality of Life

BCA's view is that even if a drug does not improve the chances of survival, it should be approved for breast cancer if it can be demonstrated to improve the quality of life for breast cancer patients. This argument, too, surfaced in the recent Avastin debate. While some patients say that they feel better on Avastin than they have on systemic chemotherapy drugs, these anecdotal reports do not amount to a systematic evaluation of the quality of life for patients on the drug. In trials where patients know that they are receiving the drug that is being evaluated, it is impossible to objectively gauge the impact of the drug on quality of life. Instead, quality of life assessments must be made in blinded trials (where the patients don't know what drug they are receiving) and must use established quality of life criteria to evaluate the results.

Since the Avastin trial that Genentech presented to the FDA was an "open label" trial, where patients knew what drug they were receiving, there was no unbiased information about quality of life available for the FDA to consider. Again, for this reason, BCA opposed approval of Avastin for breast cancer.

Less Expensive Therapies

The FDA's mission statement reads in part that the agency is "responsible for advancing the public health by helping to speed innovations that make medicines and foods more effective, safer, and *more affordable*" (emphasis added). Despite this statement, the FDA is currently prohibited by law from considering cost when it decides whether to approve new drugs for marketing or existing drugs for expanded use.

Nonetheless, with the emergence of biotech therapies being marketed at breathtaking prices, we ignore at our peril the impact of the cost of new cancer drugs on the health care system and those who are forced to rely on it. So while BCA cannot and will not argue to the FDA that it should deny approval for a drug because of cost (Avastin will reportedly cost just under $100,000 a year for breast cancer patients), we will engage with other cancer organizations, policymakers, and the drug manufacturers themselves to try to ensure that any new cancer drug that doesn't either extend life or improve the quality of life at least costs less than other treatments currently available.

Safety and Effectiveness—How Can We Tell?

Of course, none of the standards that BCA argues for in its FDA advocacy matters if the drug under consideration has not been shown to be both safe and effective. As drugs move quickly through the approval pipeline at the FDA, the challenge of assuring drug safety becomes more daunting. After all, it may take years for all the side effects of new treatments to be understood.

In the current drug approval environment, it becomes essential that the FDA follow two additional requirements in approving new treatments:

- No new treatment or expanded marketing should be approved unless at least two well-designed clinical trials have shown the benefits claimed for the drug. While this used to be required by FDA staff, more recent approvals have too often been based on a single trial. (For example, the FDA's recent approval of the use of Herceptin as monotherapy in the adjuvant setting for breast cancer was based on one-year follow-up from a single trial.)

- Any new approval of a drug should be accompanied by a requirement that the drug company conduct extensive and careful postmarketing studies and report the results to the FDA and the general public. Only with postmarketing studies will we be able to understand what a drug's long-term effects are.

We are well aware at BCA that there are many individuals and many other cancer organizations that take a different view from ours. But the stand we take is the one we believe to be in the best interests of breast cancer patients and the people who care about them. As these matters continue to be debated at the FDA and beyond, BCA will articulate its concerns about the drug approval process and work to improve it. We will also work with our many allies to make sure that the FDA has the necessary resources to protect the public's health.

May 2008

✦

The Organic Process of Activism

Think Before You Pink®, Then and Now

Way back in 2000, a close friend of mine talked to me about a conversation she had with someone doing a three-day breast cancer walk. The upshot of that conversation was a suggestion that BCA should try to determine where all the money raised in breast cancer walks was ending up. (Back then, the walks had just recently begun taking place throughout the country.) What followed from this conversation is something I call the organic process of activism, where one thing leads to the next, and a different kind of movement begins to take shape.

In response to my friend's question, we started doing some digging, and I wrote a column for the *BCA Source* titled "Exercise Your Mind" (newsletter no. 58, March–April 2000). That column turned into an op-ed in the *San Francisco Chronicle* that was picked up by other newspapers. As a result, BCA started hearing from folks all over the country who asked if BCA knew about various products being sold to raise money for breast cancer, how much money was really being donated, and where it was going.

As the questions mounted, and as more and more breast cancer cause marketing (the practice of trying to increase sales of a product by linking it to a social cause) took place, it became clear that the issue of breast cancer fund-raising practices went far beyond walks. So BCA expanded its focus. The result, in 2002, was the launch of our Think Before You Pink® campaign.

In the first year, we focused on breast cancer cause marketing in general, placing a print ad in the *New York Times*. The result was *lots* of public attention to breast cancer cause marketing. Several of the worst offenders (companies that gave mere pennies to breast cancer from their sales, or who misled the public about their efforts), including the Eureka Company (the vacuum cleaner manufacturer) and American Express, actually stopped doing this kind of marketing.

In 2003, we turned our attention for the first time to the two-timing cause-marketing companies—those that claim to care about women's lives by making a commitment to breast cancer but whose products are linked to the disease. Inspired by our allies in the environmental movement, we labeled these companies "pinkwashers." We placed another print ad in the *New York Times*, focused specifically on cosmetics companies—Avon, Revlon, Estée Lauder—that raise money for breast cancer research and support but that use chemicals in their products that have been linked to breast cancer and other health problems.

The 2003 campaign led Breast Cancer Action, in partnership with a number of other organizations and allies in the business community, to file a resolution calling on Avon shareholders to ask the company to remove harmful chemicals from its products. These efforts ultimately led to Avon agreeing to remove certain phthalates from its cosmetics and to the creation of the National Safe Cosmetics Campaign. And in 2005, California became the first state in the nation to require cosmetics companies to disclose the carcinogens and reproductive toxins in their products when it passed the Safe Cosmetics Act.

By 2004, Think Before You Pink® had become a Web-based campaign focused on the lack of coordination of breast cancer funding. With a short online animated video, we encouraged people to contact the major breast cancer research and funding agencies to work together to solve the breast cancer puzzle. Many people wrote to these entities, and the responses we received were less than reassuring, since each described itself as working with others, but in each instance in very different ways.

In 2005, the campaign returned its focus to the cause-marketing companies themselves, calling for more transparency and accountability. An online Flash video asked how much money was raised by the thousands of pink ribbon products and how much was spent marketing them. Through an online action item at ThinkBeforeYouPink .org, activists e-mailed several cause-marketing companies and asked a series of questions to help determine whether buying the product would be as good for women with breast cancer as it would be for the company.

By 2006, Think Before You Pink® was so well known that activists and reporters contacted BCA throughout the year to find out what was happening with breast cancer cause marketing. What was less clear was whether people understood who and what "pinkwashers" were, so we zeroed in on this particular set of cause marketers. We targeted car manufacturers—Ford, BMW, and Mercedes—that have breast cancer–related marketing campaigns, while at the same time manufacturing cars that emit carcinogens in their exhaust. We also generated activist e-mails to the companies through the campaign Web site.

As you can see from this issue of the *BCA Source,* our focus in 2008 is on pinkwashers again, since these companies are exposing people to toxins while claiming to care about women's lives.

By now, of course, this campaign has reached tens of thousands of people. It's been featured as a case study in effective advocacy campaigns by Fenton Communications, and ThinkBeforeYouPink.org was chosen as the Yahoo pick of the month in October 2007. It has been featured in newspapers ranging from the *New York Times* to the *Omaha World Herald* and has been a topic of discussion throughout the blogosphere.

The campaign exists and succeeds because people just like you asked for it, made it a reality, and continue to take action to address the issues that it raises. Working together, we can change the behavior of cause marketers, especially the pinkwashing companies. And when those companies change, other companies pay attention and change, too. Everyone benefits, thanks to your efforts.

September 2008

Breast Cancer Awareness Month

The Present Looks like the Past

Longtime readers of this publication know that BCA has long been critical of Breast Cancer Awareness Month (BCAM), both because of the focus on messages about "early detection" and because of the absence of information about the environmental links to breast cancer. Of course, the silence on environmental issues doesn't surprise anyone who knows the history of BCAM. That history is being replicated now in a variety of ways, none of them good for women's health.

Briefly, BCAM was created by a pharmaceutical company now called AstraZeneca (manufacturer of Arimidex and formerly of tamoxifen). The company, in addition to making drugs to treat breast cancer, has historically produced herbicides that are known carcinogens. So it's no wonder that environmental issues aren't on the agenda for official BCAM messaging.

Of course there's more to the profit cycle now, because as the incidence of breast cancer has grown, more companies have seen the wisdom of making drugs for a growing market. And they don't seem to see a problem with, at the same time, making products that might increase the risk of breast cancer. What better way to make profits than to create the disease for which you sell the treatments?

We've written in *The Source* before about Novartis, which makes the aromatase inhibitor Femara and also the herbicide Atrazine, which stimulates aromatase production in animals.

Eli Lilly is also in the game, but with an added twist. The company makes cancer drugs, including Gemzar, used to treat breast cancer. Thanks to a purchase it made last year from Monsanto, the company now also makes and markets rBGH through its subsidiary Elanco. This hormone, used to stimulate milk production in cows, had been linked to breast cancer and other cancers. To round out its profit circle Eli Lilly makes and markets Evista, a drug first approved for the treatment of osteoporosis that is also marketed to "reduce the risk of breast cancer in women at high risk of the disease" (a phrase often confused with the word *prevention*).

If you wanted to make sure that your profits were secure, you couldn't do better than to take Eli Lilly's approach: create cancer, and create the products to "prevent" and treat the disease. How perfect.

Except when it comes to the public's health, that is. Follow the money and work with BCA to end the deadly profit cycle.

Fall 2009

So Much to Celebrate,
So Much to Be Done

I have written many articles for this newsletter over many years—
first as a BCA volunteer member, then as a chair of the BCA board,
and for the past fifteen years as BCA's executive director. BCA celebrates twenty years of incredible activism this fall, and I have personally witnessed a lot of that activity. Because we tend to get so en-
grossed in the day-to-day, I think we tend to forget all that got us to
where we are today. So consider these selected highlights of BCA's
first twenty years of work.

1991   BCA founders and activists Elenore Pred, Susan
       Claymon, Belle Shayer, and Linda Reyes meet with
       the director of the National Cancer Institute (NCI) to
       demand that the NCI address the breast cancer epidemic.
       Keep in mind that 1991 is not so long ago, really.

1992   BCA helps create the California Breast Cancer Research
       Program, which has since, thanks to BCA's continued
       involvement, become a leader in involving activists and
       advocates in research and in restructuring how breast
       cancer research is funded and performed.

1993   BCA is the first organization to address the American
       Association for Advancement of Science regarding
       environmental links to breast cancer.

1996   BCA prevails in efforts to have tamoxifen added to
       California's Proposition 65 list of known and probable
       carcinogens.

1997 BCA opposes routine mammography screening of women aged forty to forty-nine. In 2010, with emerging science, BCA recommits to this position.

1998 BCA becomes the first national breast cancer organization to adopt a policy against accepting funding from companies that profit from or contribute to cancer. By 2010, BCA is the only national breast cancer organization still independent of this kind of funding.

2000 BCA leads the call to guarantee that poor and uninsured women screened for breast cancer at state expense receive prompt access to quality treatment at state expense.

2001 BCA launches the Think Before You Pink® campaign, transforming how the public and media think about cause marketing for breast cancer and how other breast cancer organizations engage in that marketing.

2002 In partnership with the Breast Cancer Fund, BCA releases the first edition of the report "State of the Evidence: What Is the Connection between the Environment and Breast Cancer?"

2003 BCA opposes the FDA's decision to allow silicone breast cancer implants back on the market.

2004 BCA leads activists at the Avon shareholder meeting, calling for the company to remove harmful chemicals from its cosmetic products. This work ultimately leads to the creation of the National Safe Cosmetics Campaign and the California Safe Cosmetics law.

2005 BCA works closely with the cities of San Francisco and Berkeley to ensure timely and effective implementation of ordinances adopting the precautionary principle of public health as a matter of local policy.

2007 Consistent with its policy of opposing pills for the prevention of breast cancer, BCA successfully opposes the STELLAR trial of raloxifene and aromatase inhibitors in healthy women.

2009 BCA activists persuade General Mills to stop using rBGH-stimulated dairy products in its pink-ribbon-

labeled Yoplait yogurt. Dannon follows suit, and now
two-thirds of the U.S. dairy market is rBGH free.

2010 BCA is one of the plaintiffs in the successful lawsuit
brought by the ACLU and the Public Patent Foundation
challenging patents on the breast cancer genes BRCA-1
and -2.

These accomplishments—and many more not listed here—are the result of an amazing amount of work by lots and lots of people, some
known and many more unknown. In a column I recently read about
the struggle for women's suffrage in the United States, the columnist
wrote: "We always need to remember that behind almost every great
moment in history, there are heroic people doing really boring and
frustrating things for a prolonged period of time."

There is still so much to do before we can declare the breast
cancer epidemic over and close BCA's doors. (After all, a cancer organization whose goal isn't to go out of business is in the wrong line
of work.) It's important to remember that all change takes long, hard
work. But there are successes along the way, and we need to celebrate
those at every opportunity.

As I prepare to hand over the reins at BCA to the next executive
director and retire from paid work at the end of 2010, I am intensely
aware of how many people have made BCA what it is today. I have
been honored to lead this fine organization, and I look forward to
seeing—and supporting—BCA's next successes.

Be well,

Barbara Brenner

Fall 2010

PART II

Thoughts on Dying and Living, 2011–2013

Thoughts on Dying and Living

Barbara had long planned to retire in 2010, at age sixty, and she and Breast Cancer Action envisioned a thorough transition period. Her retirement, in fact, came a few months early, after a number of tests indicated she most likely had ALS (amyotrophic lateral sclerosis). In March 2011, she began writing a blog, Healthy Barbs, that continued to address many of the issues she had brought up over the years in her columns for *The Source*. She continued to be critical of corporate pinkwashing, walks for various diseases, and the absence of discussion about environmental causes of cancer.

The posts were often longer and more detailed than the columns, well argued, humorous, and frequently provocative. It's likely that the title of one post aimed at the Susan G. Komen Foundation, "Gloves Off: What the Fuck, Komen?" (February 3, 2012) might have been softened before it went into the BCAction newsletter. The blog gave Barbara the freedom to take on the Komen Foundation more directly; in this post she accused the organization of being right wing and criticized its defunding of Planned Parenthood's breast cancer services. Later she would demand that its director, Nancy Brinker, resign. Barbara also drew attention to Susan Love, the noted breast cancer surgeon, and her foundation, which benefited from funding from Avon, a company that had not signed on to the Campaign for Safe Cosmetics and that continued to use known or suspected carcinogens in some of their products. Posts like these attracted many comments and testy exchanges, but Barbara seemed undeterred in calling out hypocrisy wherever she discovered it.

She continued to dissect the language of popular science writing

("Science by Press Release—Not Good News for Patients," August 26, 2011) and of health statistics ("Understanding Health Numbers," June 13, 2011). In one lucid and powerful post, "Health Activism—Not for the Faint of Heart" (September 8, 2011), Barbara described what it meant to her to be an activist—what her values were based on and how she went about her work:

> In my lexicon, an activist is someone who is clear about her/ his goals and strategic about achieving them. S/he cannot be bought—no amount of money or privileges will change her commitment to her goals. . . . The goals are about more than self-interest: they are about changing systems so many people who now suffer will benefit. More often than not, those goals and objectives are bigger than can be achieved in one lifetime, and activists know that their efforts are possible because of previous work done by others. They also know that, if they do their job right, others will come after them to advance the work. . . . Health activists have to be tough. Because they publicly take principled positions, there are always people who disagree with them and say so, sometimes in not-so-nice terms. If an activist caves because her positions have been criticized, she's not really an activist.

Barbara's toughness and commitment to her goals rarely wavered and her blog reflects that, even as her own health deteriorated and she faced daily challenges from ALS.

As always in her public career as a health activist, Barbara drew on her own experiences as a patient to explore the difficulties she and others faced in being effective advocates for themselves. "I am once again in the position of needing medical care, and too often have to struggle to get the care I need. I'm better equipped to do this than a lot of people, partly because I have so much experience being an advocate for others. When I think of what I have to do to get the best care for myself, I am deeply troubled by the fact that so few people have the resources I have that help me get what I need," she wrote in "Patient? Who's Patient?" (March 15, 2011). Over the next two years Barbara would alternate her comments on breast cancer activism with reports on her own struggle with ALS. These posts ranged from critiques of health care topics that plague our corporate and consumer society to public perceptions of ALS as Lou Gehrig's disease. She also wrote of the day-to-day challenges she faced, one of which was losing her speaking voice. At first she used a voice amplifier, then an app for her iPad called NeoKate. Kate allowed her to type what she wanted to say, then Kate would speak what had been typed ("Having a Voice, Communicating, and Somewhere in Between," June 17, 2011). In the months to come Barbara would describe the progressive losses she faced in walking and moving, along with her understanding that death was the only outcome possible. "Choices: How I Live with ALS" (March 16, 2012) offered her readers an overview of the main physical issues she had to deal with; her greatest choice in many ways was to carry her lifelong optimism with her as long as she could: "Barring a medical miracle or a tornado hitting our house, ALS will get me one day. But, until that day comes, I will work to manage what I can. Using aids like the ones I describe here enables me to continue to function at the level my energy permits. I have a lot to live for, and a lot to do. Surrender is not an option for me."

At the same time she began Healthy Barbs, Barbara also created another more private online blog for her circle of friends and family on the Web site Caring Bridge, which offers those with illnesses a way to communicate with large numbers of people. A post on May 15, 2011, was inspired by Stephen Hawking, another ALS survivor, who suggested that people with disabilities "concentrate on things your disability doesn't prevent you doing well, and don't regret the things it interferes with." Barbara wrote her first "Can and Can't List," something she would update several more times over the next year as her condition weakened. What she could do, whether enjoying music or "sleeping with my sweetie" or studying Torah, was a longer list than what she couldn't, and the can do list increased until it also included items like "enjoy the hummingbirds," "consider the wonder of the world in all its complexity," and "look for divine light." Caring Bridge cross-posted some of the Healthy Barbs pieces or referred to them but has a less formal tone. Some posts, written with her partner Susie Lampert, tell of vacations and visits to family, observations on nature and life, or share her thoughts on spirituality and religion, both of which became increasingly essential to Barbara in the months before her death.

Beginning with a teaching she offered to her synagogue, "Uncertainty, a Teaching for Rosh Hashanah 5771" (March 31, 2011, Caring Bridge), Barbara posted thoughts on Jewish celebrations and teachings on both Caring Bridge and Healthy Barbs. She had been raised in a Reform family; formal religion, including studying Torah, increasingly gave her the courage not only to fight but to accept and appreciate life with every fiber of her being. She and Susie had been involved for some years with a synagogue in Mendocino, and several talks she gave there were posted on both blog sites. In "Mi Shebeirach: Thoughts on Illness and Blessing" (October 10, 2011, Healthy Barbs) she wrote:

> Illness confronts us with some of the greatest uncertainties we ever face. In my case—and really for all of us—the uncertainty is not about what the future holds, but how it will unfold. How do we embrace illness, if that is our reality, without welcoming it? How do we continue to do what matters to us as long as we can? How do we find comfort in the support of friends and the love of God? What role does God play in a devastating illness and in healing? . . . One way for me to keep the terror in perspective is to focus on the places where God's awe is manifest. As I'm less able to get around, I notice a lot of things through the front window of our house: hummingbirds, the clouds in the sky, the quality of the light. In the right frame of mind, I draw from these things the sense of the transcendent, of the reference everywhere to God. They enable me to sense in small things the beginning of infinite significance.

Barbara's health activism had always been rooted in her belief in social justice, and those values stayed with her to the end. One of her most moving speeches, "What I Learned as a Volunteer" (December 13, 2012), given via another iPad text-to-speech app, Speak it! as she accepted the Lola Hanzel Courageous Advocacy Award from the American Civil Liberties Union of Northern California (ACLU–NC), brought multiple threads of her life together. She told the audience how important it had been to her to volunteer for the ACLU and related highlights of her time with Breast Cancer Action, emphasizing the value of creating an effective organization with integrity: "Sooner or later, all issues of social justice are connected. And we as individuals can advance the arc of history toward justice by volunteering. The world changes because we work for change."

This talk was the second-to-last post on Healthy Barbs, followed by a few more on Caring Bridge from January and February 2013 that catch the beauty of a California winter and Barbara's difficulties and great gratitude for nature and loving friends and family. Barbara's last post, "Thanks and Blessings," came on May 7, 2013. She died a few days later. Susie had promised that her obituary would read, "Barbara Brenner died after a long struggle with the breast cancer industry." Her activism illuminated her death, as it had nourished her life.

Don't Ask Me How I Am

Years ago, over lunch with a friend who had been treated for very advanced breast cancer, I asked the question many of us ask when we see people we haven't seen for a while: "How are you?" My friend very kindly responded that the question was one to which, given her situation, she couldn't possibly know the answer. Better for her if I asked "How are you today?" or "What kind of a day are you having?"

If you think about it, none of us can really know "how we are" on any given day. We can know how we feel, but not what's going on inside our bodies. For example, people who turn out to have breast cancer often feel healthy until they are told by their doctors that that lump found on their most recent mammogram is not benign.

And we can sometimes not tell by looking at someone that s/he is ill. If you look at me now, for example, I look pretty much as I always have. My hair isn't falling out, my skin tone is good, and my smile is pleasant. But I have a disease—ALS, or amyotrophic lateral sclerosis—a degenerative neurological illness for which there is no cure.

When people ask me how I am, it drives me nuts. I don't want to discuss with everyone I see what it means to live every day with a disease that I know will make me less and less functional, and ultimately kill me. How fast this will happen is unknown, but that doesn't make it easier to talk about.

What kind of a day I'm having, or how I am today, is an easier question to answer: I'm tired or not, it's easy or hard for me to walk, or I have too much going on to tell. But at least these kinds of questions don't feel as prying and insensitive as "How are you?"

Christopher Hitchens, author and journalist who has advanced esophageal cancer, recently said something, when asked how he was, that is worth remembering. He put it something like this: "I'm dying. So are you. But I'm doing it faster than you are."

I'm too busy living to spend time answering questions about my thoughts on dying. And, in any event, I don't want to discuss that topic with everyone I see. So, don't ask me how I am.

March 4, 2011

Patient? Who's Patient?

Those of you who know me know that I care deeply about words and what they convey. Years ago, not long after I became the executive director of Breast Cancer Action I had occasion to look at the derivation of the word *patient*.

The word *patient* originally meant "one who suffers." This English noun comes from the Latin word *patiens*, and the verb *patior*, meaning "I am suffering." It is related to the Greek verb *paskhein*, meaning to suffer.

Maybe it makes sense to call people who are receiving medical care "patients." After all, if they weren't suffering, they wouldn't need care, right?

But the word *suffer* has another meaning besides feeling pain or distress. It also means to tolerate or endure pain or injury, or to be at a disadvantage. If this is what it means to be a "patient," why would anyone want to be one?

No one wants to suffer—in *any* of the ways the word is defined. We particularly don't want to suffer when we're in need of medical attention. But it's quite common, I think, for people to have the hardest time getting what they need when they are not feeling well or are dealing with a medical issue. (For a great perspective on how "patients" formed a movement to change the course of history, check out Sharon Batt's *Patient No More: The Politics of Breast Cancer.*)

I am once again in the position of needing medical care, and too often have to struggle to get the care I need. I'm better equipped to do this than a lot of people, partly because I have so much experience being an advocate for others. When I think of what I have to do to get the best care for myself, I am deeply troubled by the fact that so few people have the resources I have that help me get what I need.

I think there are many things that might keep us from advocating for what we need in medical care. One thing is lack of access to care at all. But, for those of us who have health care available to us, there are a number of things that might keep us from advocating for ourselves:

- We think doctors are the experts.
- We think we don't know enough to ask the right questions.
- We're afraid that if we ask too many questions, our doctors won't like us and won't take good care of us.
- The situation in which we find ourselves is so intimidating that we are incapable of being effective advocates for ourselves.

Here's an example of what it means to advocate for oneself. I have Kaiser health insurance. Kaiser has a neurology department, but as far as I can tell, they don't have an ALS specialist. When it became clear—after many, many tests (there is no definitive test for ALS, so you have tests to rule out everything else it might be)—that I was probably dealing with ALS, I asked for a referral for a second opinion at the Forbes Norris Center in San Francisco, which specializes in ALS. That referral came easily enough, and I saw the folks at Forbes Norris twice. When I scheduled my next follow-up at Forbes Norris, I knew I would need another referral, since the first one was time limited.

So I wrote what I thought was a very nice e-mail to my doctor at Kaiser, explaining why I needed another referral and my preference for the comprehensive, coordinated care that Forbes Norris provided.

The reply I received was not encouraging. My doctor was "unable to provide" the referral I requested. She offered instead to refer me to physical and speech therapy at Kaiser, and to schedule a neurology appointment "to help with all of [my] needs."

Since this what not the answer I wanted or needed, I wrote to my

Kaiser doctor again (the e-mail system at Kaiser makes communicating with practitioners quite easy):

> As I tried to indicate in my [first] message to you, the considerable advantage to me of continuing my care at Forbes Norris is that all of the specialists who deal with ALS patients—from speech therapists, to physical therapists, to neurologists, to social workers—are all in one location, so that my limited energies and ability to move are not taxed by going to four different sites.
>
> As for a referral to physical therapy, I have had a PT work-up at Forbes Norris. I don't see why I should have to subject myself to another one. And the speech therapy referral you gave me last time was, as you suspected it would be, less than helpful. By contrast, the speech therapist at Forbes Norris is amazingly helpful.
>
> . . . Please advise to whom and how I appeal your decision not to refer me to Forbes Norris for continuing care.

The next message I got said that my doctor had forwarded the message above to her chief of staff and a new referral was on the way. My doctor apologized for the "annoyance" of having to go through this song and dance. *Annoyance* is one word for it. *Nonsense* is another.

Patient? Not I. And I suggest that those who need something from the medical system not be patient either. If you can't advocate for yourself, find someone who can advocate for you. None of us needs to suffer at the hands of the medical system. Let's find something else to call ourselves besides "patients."

March 15, 2011

Don't Make Promises You Can't Keep—
Especially in Health

You've heard or seen them: the ads or promotions for organizations promising that if you'll just support them, they will cure or eradicate any disease you care about. In ALS, it's the ALS Association promising to "create a world without ALS." That's a bold promise, since there is no effective treatment for ALS, and prevention strategies are missing in action. So where will this "world without ALS" come from?

In breast cancer in particular—and cancer in general—the promises take many forms, for example:

- An organization in Northern California calls itself Zero Breast Cancer, claiming to be "looking forward to a world without breast cancer." This goal is, to say the least, interesting, since breast cancer has been with us since ancient Greek civilization, which is where the word *cancer* comes from.

- The National Breast Cancer Coalition has "Set a Deadline for the End of Breast Cancer." If you're wondering what date to mark on your calendars, the deadline is set for January 1, 2020. This promise echoes the assurances given when the National Cancer Institute was created in 1937. The answer to cancer has always been just around the corner. It also reminds me of a time several years back that Susan Love, the famous breast cancer surgeon, announced that she would solve the breast cancer problem in ten years. When I asked her when we should start counting, she gave the answer that drives most of these kinds of promises. She said, "We start counting when we've raised all the money."

- ASCO—the American Society of Clinical Oncology and the largest organization representing cancer physicians in the world—is trying to raise money through what they are calling the Conquer Cancer Foundation, which describes itself as "committed to a world free from the fear of cancer." My read is that they want to be sure there are treatments available when people get cancer (which is where cancer docs make their profits, of course), so that cancer is a disease that is feared less, not experienced less.

- The Susan G. Komen for the Cure Foundation is "fighting every minute of every day to finish what we started and achieve our vision of a world without breast cancer." Of course, since the focus of the Komen Foundation is primarily on detection through mammography screening, it's hard to understand how we get from *fighting* cancer to a world without the disease. Also noteworthy is how Komen uses the word *cure* (they have trademarked the phrase "for the cure," and they aggressively enforce that mark). They repeatedly use the word *cure* in a context where prevention is more appropriate. For example, Komen claims that "without a cure, 1 in 8 women in the U.S. will continue to be diagnosed with breast cancer." Of course, even *with* "a cure" women will still get breast cancer—otherwise they won't need a cure.

I recognize that hope is important. But do we have to lie to people so they'll hope for the things they most desire when they or their loved ones are sick?

I cannot tell you how many people I met in my years as a breast cancer activist who believed that "the cure" was within reach, only a few years away, if we just threw more money at the problem. This was not a surprising view, given the kind of information most organizations put out about cancer. It's this kind of information, after all, that drives people to want to support cancer research.

A more rational view—one that explores the assumptions and constraints underlying cancer research and puts the cancer research effort in perspective—is hard but not impossible to find.

Really, is honesty when it comes to what can be accomplished in health really so much to ask?[1]

March 23, 2011

Note

1. Some of the sources cited in this and other posts are no longer available online. For still current links, see http://www.zerobreastcancer.org; http://www.breastcancerdeadline2020.org; http://ww5.komen.org.

Isn't It Time to Change the Message?

Those of you reading this blog are already living in the "Information Age." Seems to me that as information changes, those shifts should influence how we think about and talk about issues. Seems logical, no?

Unfortunately, this logic doesn't seem to be guiding either the Susan G. Komen for the Cure Foundation or the ALS Association, as far as I can tell. What these two organizations have in common is that they believe they are the only real players in the nonprofit world of the diseases they address. In the case of the ALS Association, they are (sadly) correct. But whether they are right on wrong on their self-perceptions, shouldn't these organizations want to help the public understand the illnesses they address? Seems to me like that's not so important to them.

Those of you who know me know I have long been interested in breast cancer and am something of an expert on the topic.

I also take a particular interest in ALS, because I now have the disease. I've been reading a number of articles recently about head injuries (often in NFL football players) that result in motor-degeneration symptoms similar to ALS, but not the same disease. What's the new information here? Well, it seems that Lou Gehrig—the mascot of the ALS Association (whose tag line reads, "Fighting Lou Gehrig's Disease")—may not have had ALS. Seems he played injured—often with concussions—and was famous for doing so.

When this news began to emerge, the chief scientific adviser for the ALS Association was quoted as saying something along the lines of, "It would be terrible to lose Lou Gehrig as a symbol of ALS, since he helps people understand what kind of disease it is."

Seems to me that if it turns out that the man on whom you have built your organization didn't have the disease that is its focus, it's time to rethink your message rather than bemoan the loss of your symbol.

The Susan G. Komen for the Cure Foundation (hereafter "Komen") seems to have a similar problem. As we have learned more and more about breast cancer, it's become clear that "early" detection with mammography only works for some women.

When Komen started—it was then called the Susan G. Komen Breast Cancer Foundation—its message was "early detection is your best prevention." That struck people who thought logically as incredibly wrong-headed, since if you were finding something "early" you certainly weren't preventing it.

That message still prevails in some communities, where young women seek mammograms because they have heard it will "prevent" breast cancer, and others are stunned to find they have a diagnosis when they recently had a mammogram.

Komen, under pressure from breast cancer activists, changed their message on mammograms to "early detection is your best protection." That's not much better, because mammograms don't protect you against breast cancer, though, *in some cases*, if combined with appropriate and timely treatment, they can protect you from dying of breast cancer.

One of the consequences of breast cancer's "popularity" is that, for some time now, there has been a great deal of money spent on research into the disease. Appropriately, some of that research has been spent on mammography screening.

As the information from those studies has emerged, it has become clear that the messages that the public has been receiving about mammograms have been so oversimplified that women both overestimate the benefits of the technology and fail to understand the limits of the concept of "early detection."

Komen has long led the way in what the public understands (and doesn't) about breast cancer. What has Komen done as this information has emerged? They've reinforced their old messages, with their leader, Nancy Brinker, arguing that it would be too confusing to women to change the message now. Interesting, coming from the person who spearheaded the confusion in the first place.

I often hear the argument that we can't discourage people from getting mammograms because, for poor women, mammography screening is often the only way they get health care. I understand this problem, but I don't think we can let all of our conversations and understanding of breast cancer rest on mammography's shoulders. The real issue for poor women and all people who are medically underserved is *access* to comprehensive, affordable health care. These folks are as entitled as the rest of us to messages about health that take into account the information available.

Oversimplifying is dangerous, especially when information is available that would help people understand better the diseases that affect or may someday affect them.

March 28, 2011

Uncertainty, a Teaching for
Rosh Hashanah 5771

Barbara gave this teaching at our synagogue in Mendocino, California, as she was facing the prospect of what is now a reality. We thought you would enjoy reading it.

Barbara and Susie

I was in Ashland at the Oregon Shakespeare Festival when Rabbi Margaret asked me to prepare a reflection (or something like one) for this afternoon. So Shakespeare was on my mind, as are so many other things as I prepare to retire from my job as a full-time change agent in the world of breast cancer and as I confront what seems to be a medical condition that is hard to define. So I guess you could say that the theme of this reflection is change and uncertainty and how we deal with them.

Maybe the only thing that's not uncertain about change is that it's inevitable. You probably know that. But it seems to me that change happens to us in ways we expect (like Rosh Hashanah or choosing to have a child), in ways we don't expect (like illness or accident), and in ways we work to make happen (like going on a weight loss diet or, in my case, pushing for changes in cancer policy).

What's less inevitable is how we respond to the changes we don't anticipate: we can embrace them; we can be paralyzed by them; we can learn from them; and, sometimes, we can respond in all these ways at the same time.

All change brings uncertainty. Some types of uncertainty are worse than others. The uncertainty that accompanies the possibility of having a dreaded disease ranks in my world among the worst of all. When I was diagnosed with breast cancer at the age of forty-one, I quickly learned that there was little I could do to change the outcome of my illness. I've had all the treatments, and time will tell. So all that there was to do to affect that outcome, I did.

Then I found myself thinking about the hundreds of thousands of women who would be diagnosed after I was, and what might be done to create a more certain future for them and a different future for the generation of women and men that will follow after them. These thoughts led me to my work as a breast cancer activist.

I have done this work for fifteen years. I know that my activism has taught me a great deal. Keeping my ears and heart open to the many wonderful—and some not-so-wonderful—people I've met doing this work has fueled my work to change the direction of breast cancer treatment and prevention. I can honestly say that I have had an impact—on the lives of people I've touched over the years and on the policy decisions that are being made about cancer in this country and beyond. Now that I've announced my retirement, people I don't even know are writing to thank me for things that I did, some of which I don't even remember doing. It's touching, and a little embarrassing.

One of the reasons it's a little embarrassing is that no one works alone, and often people with the biggest mouths or those sitting in the chair nearest the camera get the most credit for the work done by many, many people.

Reflecting on fifteen years of activism has reminded me that the kind of change that we work to make happen takes a long time, often longer than we have the time or energy for. So deciding to step aside so others can lead leaves me thinking about the uncertainty of what lies ahead for the things I have spent so much of my life working on: the work of challenging people's assumptions, getting them to think in new ways about things they think they already know, and inspiring them to act in a way that will have benefits for all of us.

Uncertainty is no small thing. Shakespeare said it best in *Hamlet*. Hamlet makes a famous speech in Act III that starts out, "To be, or not to be." But the part that actually talks about uncertainty comes later on and goes like this:

> But that the dread of something after death,
> The undiscover'd country from whose bourn
> No traveller returns, puzzles the will,
> And makes us rather bear those ills we have
> Than fly to others that we know not of?
> Thus conscience does make cowards of us all,
> And thus the native hue of resolution
> Is sicklied o'er with the pale cast of thought,
> And enterprises of great pitch and moment
> With this regard their currents turn awry
> And lose the name of action.

I saw *Hamlet* twice recently at the Oregon Shakespeare Festival, but this quote had been sent to me several years ago by a young woman named Julia. Julia's breast cancer had been misdiagnosed for a long time, and by the time it was found, her disease was very far advanced. Julia is an artist, and the action she took was to turn her experience into a very powerful exhibit of photographs about what it means to be Julia. I met her at a symposium at which we were both presenting talks on the ethics of breast cancer. We made a fast connection and spent many hours talking, first in person, then by e-mail and phone, since we live on opposite sides of the country.

Julia is not yet forty, and she has two preteenage daughters. She wrote to me recently that she has decided to stop treatment for her advanced breast cancer and accept palliative care. She wrote: "I feel like I have made the right choice. And, as Bernard Shaw says, 'the world belongs to the masters of reality.'"

For Julia, this change in her life is about both learning from and embracing change in the face of great uncertainty about not what the future holds but how it will unfold for her.

In the words of Shakespeare, it seems to me that Julia has not let her will be puzzled by the dread of something after death. And I think that maybe, just maybe, it's that kind of courage that gets each of us through another day, and—God willing—another year. Keeping our eyes open in the face of uncertainty is one important way to not lose the name of action.

March 31, 2011

A New Name

I decided recently that I wanted to take a Hebrew name (I didn't get one at birth), so I contacted my friend Rabbi Margaret Holub of the Mendocino Coast Jewish Community and asked for some advice about how best to go about this process.

Rabbi Margaret responded enthusiastically and over several weeks/months helped guide my search for the perfect Hebrew name for me. During the course of our conversation, she told me a story that I love, so here it is: there is a practice among some Jewish people with life-threatening illnesses to change their names to fool the angel of death. Sounded like a great idea to me, and I didn't even know that when I decided to take a Hebrew name.

So today, Wednesday, April 6, we had a little ceremony at the San Francisco Mikvah Israel B'nai David to "officially" confer that name on me. A mikvah is a ritual purification bath used by Jews for millennia to commemorate certain occasions. There is no formal "naming" ceremony for adults, because most names are given at birth, so we made one up.

Present today (actually, or in spirit) were the rabbi, me, Susie (of course), and a very small number of very dear friends. The ceremony involved Margaret's explaining the function of the mikvah, friends' sharing their thoughts about this moment of transition for me, and my thoughts about choosing the name.

Margaret's explanation of the function of the mikvah was very helpful. As she put it in an e-mail message she sent in preparation for the ceremony:

"One way I understand immersing in a mikvah (a pool of 'living

water') is that it has to do with moving from whatever is one's present
state into a state of heightened holiness, openness, blessing, presence. . . . Going into the water, 'the womb and the grave,' is thus a kind
of rebirth. A way that I learned from my beloved teacher to make this
shift is to form an intention for the state one hopes to move toward."

My friends who were gathered had lovely and very moving
things to say about this journey of life we are all on together.

Then I used a speech synthesizer program to "read" what I had
written about my choice of the name Shefa. Here's what I had to say:

> I was born as the third child in what became a large Reform
> Jewish family. None of us was given a Hebrew name, though
> all four boys in my family were bar mitzvahed, and all of us
> were confirmed in the Jewish faith.
>
> At a family wedding recently, I noticed that the proud
> father of the groom—who is also my younger brother Mark—
> was referred to by a Hebrew name. I asked him how he came
> to have one. He told me he had chosen one for himself some
> years ago.
>
> Reflecting on my experience with aliyot (the honor of
> being called to the Torah) at the Mendocino Coast Jewish
> Community, and facing an unwished-for journey with ALS, I
> began thinking about new ways to relate to the world and to
> God, and to my faith as a Jew. I contacted Rabbi Margaret to
> ask her to work with me in choosing a Hebrew name.
>
> In our exploration, I resonated with words that conveyed
> concepts of dawn and connection, but kept searching for the
> name that fit me.
>
> In the midst of these discussions and ruminations, I
> made a trip to Yosemite, which is for me one of those places
> where God's presence is manifest. I spent some time at Lower
> Yosemite Falls, watching the drops of water from the falls
> tumble down the creek to the Merced River, flowing through
> all of creation. Watching made me think about how I am like a
> drop of water, connected to and part of the abundance of God's
> creation.

My intention—my kavvanah—is to find my way to a place that lets me connect to the abundance of God's creation, and to the source of it. This intention is reflected in the name I have chosen. Shefa means "abundance."

Then I took the requisite shower (you have to be *very* clean to get into a mikvah—I had showered twice today even *before* we went to the mikvah) and joined my friends who were gathered around the mikvah pool itself. I walked down the steps in the very warm water and prepared to completely immerse myself under the water, and to do so three times.

Unfortunately, the first time I immersed, I inhaled water, which led to a scary moment of choking. But with the loving support of my friends, I calmed down from that and proceeded to dunk (omitting my head from the process) the requisite three times. After each time, I recited a prayer (with the rabbi's help, of course).

Then I got out of the mikvah, wrapped in a towel, and Rabbi Margaret read a passage about the name Shefa. Then all my friends put their hands on me, and the rabbi said a blessing giving me the name Shefa. We all sang a Shehecheyanu (a prayer thanking God for bringing us to this moment). Then it was time for me to get dressed.

We gathered again in the little anteroom at the mikvah and shared a kiddush that Margaret supplied and led.

It was a remarkable afternoon, filled with love and intention and a connection to the holy places that are in all of our lives, especially when we connect deeply with people we love.

On the way home from the mikvah, we picked up our favorite dessert from Mission Pie to celebrate. It's a walnut pie night!

April 6, 2011

Passover

Hello, dear family and friends,
     We are back from a very quick trip to Montreal. We made the journey so Barbara could give feedback to the National Film Board of Canada about a breast cancer documentary currently in production. Barbara was interviewed for the film last fall, and we were both very excited to see the emerging work and to be with the fabulous people who are making this documentary. Stay tuned for more information on the film. We'll tell what we can as soon as it's ready to be released.

     We came home quickly from Montreal because, as those of you who are Jewish (and many who aren't) probably know, Passover (or Pesach) starts tomorrow at sundown with the Seder meal and service. As we have done for many years, we are hosting a Seder at our home this year but, because of the changes in our lives, have felt the need both to reduce the number of people attending and to ask some of the participants to do more to help prepare the meal than we have in years past. Everyone who was asked to pitch in has responded generously, and we're looking forward to the day of preparation and the evening that follows.

     We (mostly Susie) have also been thinking about what we celebrate at Passover and have decided to rework our Seder service to reflect more of what that celebration means to us now, at this stage of our lives. The story of Passover is, traditionally, the story of the Exodus of the Jews from oppression in Egypt, led by Moses. It is a story of transformation from slavery to freedom. But transformation takes many forms, so we are asking ourselves and our guests to think about and focus on the transformation in their lives in the past few years:

whether they be about new relationships, job changes, or, in our case, retirement from work and confronting the challenges of increasing disability. And we will also focus on what form happiness takes for each of us, as we look forward to another year filled with many things that make each of us happy.

We wish for you, and for everyone in the world, a happy Passover and a year filled with positive transformation and many happy moments.

Our Seder last night was a fabulous evening for so many reasons: the people we love who attended, the work that we had done to revise our Haggadah, and the focus on transformation and joy that we all brought to the Seder service.

Susie and I are, of course, affected differently by my ALS diagnosis, and we addressed it in different ways in the part of the Seder where everyone talked about transformations they had experienced or are experiencing now.

We thought you'd be interested in our reflections from the Seder, so here they are.

Susie: Over the past year, I have had many delightful transitions: I retired from paid work, I turned sixty, and I started volunteering at the Magic Theatre. And then, just as everything was looking so positive, Barbara and I were faced with this new challenge of her health. In that light, the transformation I'm pursuing now is learning to accept help and to see that not as surrender but instead as liberation.

Barbara: *Webster's* dictionary defines *transformation* as an act, process, or instance of change in structure, appearance, or character. A conversion, revolution, makeover, alteration, or renovation. My transformation over the past year would fit many of these definitional words. I retired from fifteen years of full-time breast cancer activism and transformed into a blogger activist.

I was diagnosed with an illness that will rob me of my ability to speak, walk, and ultimately to move and began to transform my life into one that I can lead from a more limited frame than I'm used to. In that context, I have begun to explore my Jewish faith more deeply and transformed into a woman with a Hebrew name and one who is happily studying the Torah.

While I don't look forward to what my diagnosis will bring, I am anticipating with interest the continuing transformations that will accompany the continuing changes in my life.

In our Seder service, as we opened the door for Elijah, we read this selection from "Open Door" in *A Field Guide to Getting Lost,* by Rebecca Solnit:

> Leave the door open for the unknown, the door into the dark. That's where the most important things come from, where you yourself came from, and where you will go. Three years ago I was giving a workshop in the Rockies. A student came in bearing a quote from what she said was the pre-Socratic philosopher Meno. It read, "How will you go about finding that thing the nature of which is totally unknown to you?" ... The things we want are transformative, and we don't know or only think we know what is on the other side of that transformation. Love, wisdom, grace, inspiration—how do you go about finding these things that are in some ways about extending the boundaries of the self into unknown territory, about becoming someone else? ...
>
> The important thing is not that Elijah might show up someday. The important thing is that the doors are left open to the dark every year. Jewish tradition holds that some questions are more significant than their answers, and such is the case with this one. ... For it is not, after all, really a question about whether you can know the unknown, arrive in it, but how to go about looking for it, how to travel.

Thanks to Rabbi Margaret Holub, of the Mendocino Coast Jewish Community, for giving us a copy of the Solnit essay as we prepared for Passover and our contemplation of journeys from the known to the unknown, from the present to the future.

We wish everyone a wonderful Passover, filled with love and transformation.

April 17–19, 2011

There's That Person with . . .

I'm "meeting" some wonderful people as I deal with ALS, including folks who have other conditions that impair their ability to function in some way. Most of these meetings are by e-mail, but they are delightful nonetheless.

I was listening recently on my local PBS station—KQED—to a radio perspective recorded by Patty, who has Parkinson's disease. Fortunately, medication for now controls for Patty some of the movement challenges that that disease presents. In that commentary, she talked, among other things, about being concerned that by going public with her disease she would become "that person with Parkinson's."

We All Have Something

Most of us have—or will have at some point—some condition that will make us "that person with . . ." When I was executive director of Breast Cancer Action, I was concerned that people would see me and say to themselves, "Here comes that breast cancer person again."

Of course, breast cancer people can identify each other by those damn pink ribbons or pink wristbands, or the chemotherapy-induced baldness or head turbans, or the more direct Cancer Sucks buttons that tell the real story of a breast cancer diagnosis.

Other conditions are not so easily identified as you walk down the street or sit in a coffee shop. When I see people who have trouble walking or hear people having trouble speaking, I can't tell what the underlying problem is, but—because I now share these characteristics—I'm far more sympathetic than I used to be.

None of us wants to be identified as the illness we have. We are all human beings, with thoughts, and feelings, and emotions, things we want to do and are doing, and things to contribute to the world. Patty, for instance, is dancing!

Technology: Part of the Answer

I'm being public by blogging and tweeting, but that has a limited audience. Pretty soon (no telling when), I won't be reminding people about ALS by the way I walk or talk, because I won't be doing either, and certainly not doing them in public.

Technology is making many things possible for people like me. I have a program called Speak it! on my iPad that translates the words I type into audible voice. There's another program, called NeoKate, that supposedly works the same way, but I haven't figured out how to use it yet. And there's a somewhat expensive program called JayBee that has prepared phrases that make it easy to make audible what you want to say, even if you can't talk. That program doesn't run on the iPad.

These are just a few examples. There are many more programs available for people, some for folks who can no longer type because they have lost control of the muscles in their hands.

What We Can't See Is Still a Problem

I'm left with this question: how important is it to be public about what we have so that the communities in which we live will know that there is something going on that is causing their neighbors to suffer in some way? Or so that people will think about whether there are things they can do that might help others who are struggling?

ALS, unlike breast cancer, is not a public disease, because the people who have it almost inevitably end up confined to their homes or nursing homes. They don't go out, either because they can't physically manage to or they are too self-conscious to be seen in such a compromised situation.

But we need to pay attention to what we can't see, as well as to what we can.

So if you have friends with some illness or condition that makes it hard for them to be in the public eye, think about what it means to them, and to us as a society. Maybe we should find ways to help make those people visible and able to continue to be their full human selves, and maybe be less self-conscious than they otherwise would be.

April 26, 2011

The Obligation of Privilege

I am a person of privilege. I am well educated, I know how to get the things I need, and I have the resources at my disposal to get them, usually. Privilege means having access and knowing you have it.

Being a person of privilege doesn't keep people from getting sick—at least, not always—but it can sure help deal with the consequences of being ill.

For me, the obligation of privilege is to pay it forward: to do all I can to make sure that the benefits that I get are available to others in need, and to articulate my advantages in ways that make it clear that they reflect injustices that we as a society must address.

My topic this week is about privilege in health care. But I think you can see from the analysis below that privilege is a reality in all aspects of our lives and needs to be addressed in all of them.

Privilege in the Politics of Health Care

Many Republicans are privileged. In a recent *New York Times* survey, people were asked whether it's the government's job to provide health care for the poor. Seventy-one percent of the Republicans surveyed said no. But asked whether the government is responsible for providing health care for the elderly, 55 percent of Republicans said yes. Seems that Republicans can see themselves getting old—and entitled to government-sponsored health care if they do. They just can't see themselves as poor.

I think most Republicans are, like me, people of privilege. One big difference between me and them is that they seem mostly—at least as far as this survey reveals—to think that their privilege doesn't carry with it any obligations.

Stories of Privilege in Cancer

My story: When I was diagnosed with breast cancer, the word spread pretty fast among my community of friends. My friend Carol called to suggest I see a certain surgeon. I had already called that surgeon's office, but he was booked for many weeks into the future. So imagine my surprise when I got a call from my partner, Susie, saying that I had an appointment with that surgeon for six o'clock that very evening.

When I inquired later about how that appointment had miraculously appeared, I learned that Carol had a friend—Muffie—who was one of our city's great movers and shakers. (Muffie tragically died of brain cancer last year at the age of fifty-nine.) Muffie called the surgeon's academic boss at the University of California–San Francisco. She told UCSF emphatically that I needed to see the surgeon and that they had better pay attention because I was the lawyer for the Speaker of the California Assembly, which had a lot to say about funding for the university.

I was, of course, deeply grateful for the effort that my friends had made on my behalf at the same time that I was intensely aware that this is not the way the world should work. People who need to see doctors should be able to see them without the intervention of powerful friends.

I never forgot the kind of care and support I got when I had breast cancer, and I used every opportunity given to me as I led Breast Cancer Action to articulate the need for everyone to have that kind of care.

Lance Armstrong's story: Everyone knows this story, I think. Lance Armstrong was diagnosed with late-stage testicular cancer. Through the miracle of modern medicine and the strength of his incredibly athletic body, he recovered from cancer and went on to win the Tour de France.

But have you ever heard Lance say one word about all the access he had to the best care, thanks in no small part to who he is and the resources he had? I have always wondered why Armstrong has never used his considerable influence to advance the needs of all cancer patients to get the kind of care he got—though I have seen lots of ads of Armstrong promoting drugs made by Bristol-Myers-Squibb, the company that made *his* very expensive cancer drugs.

Jerri Nielsen FitzGerald's story: Jerri Nielsen wasn't as famous as Lance Armstrong, but she had her moment in the sun. She's the doctor who, in 1999, stuck on the South Pole where she was working, did a biopsy on herself and then had chemotherapy drugs airlifted to the South Pole. Later she was airlifted out of the South Pole. Both the drug drop and her airlift out were enormously expensive. Dr. Nielsen was very grateful. She wrote a book about her experience, called *Ice Bound: A Doctor's Incredible Battle for Survival at the South Pole* (later turned into a movie starring Susan Sarandon). And until her death from breast cancer at the early age of fifty-seven, she traveled the world as a motivational speaker.

But she never talked about the resources used to help her or how we might allocate resources to make sure everyone has the care they need.

A Story of Privilege in ALS

As readers of this blog know, I have ALS, an insidious, pernicious, and unrelenting disease that is already making it hard for me to walk and will one day put me in a wheelchair. In order to stay in our three-story home of thirty-six years once I am unable to walk, we will have to install an elevator. One aspect of privilege is that we have the financial resources to cover the cost of this change. Another is subtler, and that has to do with getting permission from the city planning authorities to make this addition.

Putting in an elevator means changes to the footprint of our house to accommodate the machine plus the room we will need for a caretaker. Changing the footprint of the house means we need permission to do something the zoning code says we can't do. This is called a variance. In San Francisco, you have to apply to the city for a variance, and there is a somewhat involved process for getting your application heard and approved.

We were told by many people that this process could take

months, and we don't have months, given the progressive nature of my illness. But as privileged people do, we have friends. Some of our friends are people who understand the approval process and how to move it forward. So thanks to these friends and the responsiveness of city employees to our situation, our application for a variance moved forward with what we hear is record speed.

We are, of course, deeply grateful for the help we are getting from all quarters as we work to stay in our home, but we are intensely aware that there must be others similarly situated who do not have the access we do to get what they need. We know we are no more deserving than these people and that the system needs to pay attention to their needs when they arise.

So once our construction is well under way, we will work with San Francisco city officials to make sure that the process for applying for a variance when disability is the cause is clear and understandable to everyone who needs it. That's our obligation as people of privilege.

May 4, 2011

Can and Can't List

It's ALS Month, and the newspapers are carrying stories about survivors. The most famous survivor, I think, is Stephen Hawking, who has been living with ALS for forty-eight years. Though he is now completely paralyzed and speaks through a computer, he continues to work. In an interview with the *New York Times* on Tuesday, May 10, Dr. Hawking advised others with ALS and other disabilities to "concentrate on things your disability doesn't prevent you doing well, and don't regret the things it interferes with. Don't be disabled in spirit, as well as physically."

This is great advice. Easier to follow, I imagine, if you're not in the midst of losing the abilities you've previously had. In thinking about this, I decided it might help me to do a can/can't list, and maybe update it periodically. Here's my first crack at it. It will change—that's the nature of a progressive disease.

CAN	CAN'T
PLAY PIANO, ENJOY BEAUTIFUL MUSIC	sing
WRITE, TYPE FAST	talk without a voice amplifier; proofread well (though this is not an ALS effect)
THINK	express my thoughts well in spoken words
WALK	walk fast or far, run, or hike

READ	read out loud very well
SLEEP WITH MY SWEETIE	sleep on my back
MOVE	move fast
SIT CROSS-LEGGED ON THE FLOOR	balance standing on one leg (but I couldn't before ALS, either)
DO *NYT* CROSSWORD PUZZLES	except for Thursday mostly, Friday, or Saturday (but I couldn't before ALS)
EAT SOME FOODS I LOVE	eat and talk at the same time; eat certain foods
EAT ALL THE ICE CREAM I WANT (maintaining weight is important for ALS patients)	
CHOP FRUIT AND VEGETABLES AND MAKE GREAT CHICKEN AND TUNA SALAD	help clean up the kitchen late in the evening
ENGAGE IN SOME SOCIAL ACTIVITY (but not as much as I used to because it's both hard and tiring for me)	
TALK, IF I DO IT SLOWLY AND NOT TOO MUCH AND NOT TOO LATE IN THE DAY AND NOT WHEN I'M EATING	engage in verbal banter
LAUNDRY	

May 15, 2011

❦

That's Why They Call Them "Trials"

Given the times we seem to be in, maybe you're thinking you're about to read a blog about the trials and tribulations of Donald Trump, who can't seem to tear himself away from the big bucks of an NBC contract to run for president; or the upcoming trial of Dominique Strauss-Kahn, managing director of the International Monetary Fund, on rape charges; or the struggles of Maria Shriver, who turns out to have been married to another male politician who can't seem to keep his pants zipped.

While those topics are undoubtedly more fun to explore, they are not my subject today. I want to address the serious topic of drug clinical trials, a topic that most people who aren't doctors—and, tragically, some who are—don't understand.

What Is a Drug Clinical Trial?

Clinical trials are used to advance scientific research into the treatment of illnesses.

A clinical trial is a medical research process used to determine if a drug is (1) safe for humans to take; and (2) effective to treat the medical condition that it is intended to address. The drug under investigation—called the treatment—is compared to what is called a "control," which is either a placebo (a pill or infusion that looks like the drug under investigation but that has no biological properties) or an existing treatment for the condition, so that researchers can determine whether the drug under investigation is more effective than the alternative to which it's being compared. The treatment group of patients and the control group of patients have to be balanced in number so that the results of the trial are meaningful.

Drug trials are necessary because without them there is no way of knowing whether the treatment drug that is the subject of the trial will work for the patients in the trial.

There are a couple of other features of well-designed trials that are important to try to ensure that the outcomes of the trial reflect how the drug being tested works, rather than any sort of bias on the part of those administering the trial. These features are "randomization" and "blindness."

Randomization is the process by which patients in the trial are assigned to receive either the drug under investigation or the control. By assigning patients at random, researchers avoid any bias that might creep into trial results by choosing, for example, the apparently healthier patients to receive the drug or the less healthy patients to receive the control.

Blindness refers to who knows what about which patients are in which group—the treatment group or the control group. Ideally, drug trials are "double blind," meaning that neither the researchers nor the patients know which group the patient is in. Double-blind trials keep researchers from making judgments about how patients are doing based on what they are known to be taking. They may also keep patients from deciding to drop out of trials because they didn't get into the treatment group. (Open-label trials—where both the patients and the researchers know what drug is assigned—have become much more common in breast cancer than double-blind trials.)

A drug trial is considered a success if the patients getting the treatment drug do better than patients in the control group by a statistically significant percentage. A successful trial tells nothing about whether the treatment drug actually worked in an individual patient. After all, it's possible that the patient would have improved without the drug in question. Miracles do sometimes happen in medicine and not necessarily because doctors make them happen.

Clinical Trials in the Abstract

I know a lot about clinical trials from my work as a breast cancer activist. From that work, I have come to believe that trials should demonstrate that the drug being tested can do at least one of three things before it is marketed to the public:

- improve survival
- improve quality of life
- cost less than existing, equally effective treatments

These ideas about the goals and structures of clinical trials are fine in the abstract. It's harder when they have very personal implications, either for you or for someone you love. While no promises are ever made to patients entering clinical trials, it's hard for the patients or the people who love them to not believe at some level that the drug under investigation will improve their lives. People often enter trials believing this, no matter what they are told about the purpose of the trial.

The Personal Side

That my friends share this belief was evident when I told them that I was being screened to see if I'm eligible to be in a clinical trial. Many have hoped for me that if I was eligible for the trial, I would get the drug being investigated, not the control, which in this case is a placebo. That hope seems to convey the belief that the drug will work. Whether it will or not is, in fact, what the trial is intended to test.

I know that participating in a clinical trial means taking a chance that I won't get the drug under investigation, as well as the chance that that drug won't work anyway. I know that it's impossible to know from a clinical trial whether the drug under investigation will advance the knowledge of what does and doesn't work to treat ALS.

And I'll also keep in mind, as I enter the trial, that placebos also work sometimes.

May 19, 2011

People's Lives as the Endpoints of Medical Research— Now There's a Nifty Idea

A Little History, from a Breast Cancer Perspective

During my time at Breast Cancer Action, I became something of an expert on reading clinical trial data. I learned that the success of clinical trials is based on what scientists call "the primary endpoint." That's the effect of the drug under study on what the scientists are trying to study.

And, during that time, the primary endpoint of many studies shifted from "overall survival" (OS)—did the people in the study live longer?—to "progression-free survival" (PFS)—did it take longer for the cancer to grow in people in the study receiving the study drug, as compared to the control group?

Why did this shift take place?

It seems logical that if it takes longer for cancer to grow, the people with the cancer will live longer. And both people with cancer and drug companies are impatient for results, though for different reasons. People with cancer want drugs today that don't have so many side effects and that help them live longer. Drug companies want to get their drugs approved quickly so they can capture a share of the big markets, and cancer is a very big market.

With most types of cancer, you have to study a lot of people for a long time to figure out if the treatment you're giving helps them live longer. The thinking behind the shift in primary endpoints of studies, motivated by impatience, was this: we can determine whether a drug affects PFS more quickly than whether it extends OS.

And if PFS indicates that a drug will work to extend the lives of cancer patients, then we can get to the market faster. Viewed this way, PFS is a "surrogate"—a stand-in—for OS, and studying it is just as good as studying OS.

The Rub

Unfortunately, it turns out that delaying progression of cancer doesn't predict very well whether a person with the cancer will survive longer.

In the case of Avastin, a drug made by Genentech and approved for several cancers, the attempt to keep approval for its use in breast cancer has, at least so far, been foiled by the fact that in no study has Avastin been shown to improve overall survival of breast cancer patients, though it does delay progression.

The FDA is still considering whether to withdraw Avastin from the breast cancer market. The stakes are very high for Genentech, but they are higher for people like you and me.

The Lesson

The reason the stakes of the Avastin issue are high for folks like us is that we need drugs that actually help us when we're sick, not ones that may control some biological element related to our disease but don't really make us better. And we sure don't need any more drugs that make us feel awful (that is, degrade our quality of life) while not helping us at all. We are the ones who take these drugs and need them to work in a way that actually helps us. The use of surrogate endpoints puts too much emphasis on the "surrogate" and not enough on the people—us—the drugs are supposed to be helping.

Surrogate Endpoints: They're Not Just for Cancer

There was a story you might have missed in the news in the past week—what with all the items about tornadoes and debt limits and other scary things—about using drugs to raise "good cholesterol" in the hopes that, like lowering bad cholesterol, doing so would extend the lives of people with heart disease.

In this case, the surrogate endpoint was a measurable increase in "good cholesterol," on the theory that if that goes up, your heart is healthier.

The drug used to raise good cholesterol is niacin. It's apparently pretty hard to tolerate—patients report flushing and headaches. And the drug did indeed raise good cholesterol, but it didn't do a thing to improve the heart health of the people taking it. The surrogate endpoint was a failure.

When it comes to ALS, the disease with which I'm now dealing, the causes and biological drivers are not understood, so there are as yet no real surrogates to try to control with drugs. ALS drugs that get tested will have to improve people's symptoms, actually delay their decline in function (this is meaningful delayed progression, which improves quality of life), or help them live longer. I think that's a good thing.

Can We Focus More on People?

Maybe it's time to take a step back from the rush to approve drugs as fast as possible and make sure they work for people who are suffering, no matter what the condition being addressed. After all, we're not surrogate endpoints; we're human beings.

June 3, 2011

Understanding Health Numbers

Not Easy, but Important

T he twenty-first century seems to be, among other things, the Age of Health. Everybody's concerned about health, everyone's talking about health, and every cultural medium is flooded with ads about how to improve your health. The idea seems to be that if you're smart enough and take enough of the right drugs, you'll live forever.

Whether you believe that myth or not, the ability to read and understand numbers in medical studies is becoming increasingly important. I've been talking about this for years, starting with the study of tamoxifen (a breast cancer treatment drug) for use in healthy women to reduce their risk of developing (not "preventing") breast cancer.

The "Tamoxifen for Prevention" Story

In 1998, when the study results were announced to great fanfare, the scientific journals and press reports breathlessly reported that women taking tamoxifen reduced their chances of getting breast cancer by a stunning 50 percent. Reading this information, women naturally concluded that if they took tamoxifen, they could reduce their individual risk of developing breast cancer by almost 50 percent. From the hoopla that characterized and surrounded this news, you'd think we had finally cured cancer. Not really.

The 50 percent number led to the wrong conclusion. It turned out that for individual women, the amount they would reduce their risk by taking tamoxifen was actually 2 percent. What's the difference? The difference is between "relative" and "absolute" risk reduction.

A Brief Digression: Risk Reduction Is Not Prevention

Before I get into the numbers and unravel the difference between relative and absolute risks or benefits, a few words about words. The tamoxifen study—like many subsequent studies of other drugs like raloxifene (Evista) and exemestane (Aromasin)—was described as a breast cancer prevention study. Its official name was BCPT-1: Breast Cancer Prevention Trial 1. And the results were described in terms of how much breast cancer was prevented. But some people in the study who took tamoxifen *got* breast cancer, just not as many as people who didn't take the drug. So for any individual woman, tamoxifen and other drugs used for the same purpose *reduce the risk* of getting breast cancer. They do not *prevent* the disease. The general understanding of the word *prevention* is that if you do step A, you will not get disease B. When scientists and health policy people use the word *prevention* to mean anything else, they mislead and confuse people. That shouldn't be the goal, should it?

It's Absolutely about You

The difference between "relative" and "absolute" benefit or risk is important to understand. I know that from my work as a breast cancer activist. I also know it because the *New York Times,* in an article published in the Science section on May 30, 2011, reported that "Translation Matters in Choices on Data." The article describes the different ways that the same medical data can be presented and talks about how important it is to clearly present data so people can understand it. Since the *New York Times* reported it, this information must matter, right?

There are basically three different ways to convey information about a study of a drug to reduce the risk of a disease: relative risk reduction, absolute risk reduction, and number needed to treat.

In the simplest possible terms, here's the difference among these three ways of describing the numbers, using a hypothetical example.

When someone says that taking a drug reduces your risk of disease by half, that's a relative risk reduction number.

Another way to convey exactly the same information is to say that the risk of the disease is 2 percent for people who don't take the drug, but your risk if you take the drug is reduced to 1 percent. Your risk has been reduced by half, but in absolute terms that's a reduction of only 1 percent. In other words, in this hypothetical 98 percent of people won't get cancer if they don't take the drug; but if everyone takes the drug, that number changes to 99 percent.

A third way to convey exactly the same information is to say that one hundred people would have to be treated with the drug for one person to get the benefit of the risk reduction from it. This number matters a lot if you're concerned (or should be) about the other effects the drug might have, which are referred to medically as "side" effects.

For a real-life example, we can look at these kinds of numbers from the tamoxifen prevention trial. In that study, as mentioned above, the relative risk reduction was 49 percent. The absolute risk reduction was 2.1 percent. The number needed to treat to prevent one case of breast cancer was forty-eight.

So when a medical professional recommends you start a drug, you should start by asking what your risk is if you don't take the drug and what your risk will become if you take the treatment. And what are the potential side effects?

"Other Effects": The Devil's in the Details

All drugs have side effects. Any drug powerful enough to prevent a serious disease like cancer is going to have other effects on your health besides potentially reducing your risk of getting cancer. With tamoxifen, the most serious risk is endometrial cancer. The drug also increases the risk of stroke, deep vein thrombosis (blood clots), and cataracts. Many women also experience hot flashes and vaginal discharge with tamoxifen.

The risks of the other effects, and their seriousness, will depend a lot on the individual to whom the drug is offered and that person's current medical condition. But in almost every case where we're giving strong drugs to people to reduce their risk of getting sick, the "other effects" can loom very large, indeed.

Pay Attention to How Numbers Are Reported

The take-home message in the *New York Times* article on how reporting data matters is this: "Journalists have to be careful about press releases with 'new' or 'groundbreaking' studies presented with relative risk reductions." I would add that scientists should be required by the journals that publish their studies to report the absolute risk reduction numbers, as well as the number needed to treat.

Tamoxifen Redux: Aromatase Inhibitors for Breast Cancer "Prevention"

In the early 2000s, I was attending a San Antonio Breast Cancer Symposium where the first data on an aromatase inhibitor (AI) for treating breast cancer were presented. There was a great deal of excitement about the data. It was the kind of excitement that meant that medical practice was about to change, and did it ever. Almost overnight, oncologists began prescribing an AI called Arimidex (anastrozole) for postmenopausal women with hormone-receptor-positive breast cancer.

Up to this point, the standard treatment in this setting had been tamoxifen. But the news of the AI study was so striking that doctors came up to me at the San Antonio meeting to assure me that tamoxifen was dead.

Tamoxifen's obituary hadn't really been written at the time and still hasn't. But the other thing that I heard at that San Antonio meeting was from advocates and activists who were concerned that this new class of drugs would be tested in healthy women for breast cancer risk reduction, just as tamoxifen had been.

Those advocates were right. At a huge cancer meeting recently in Chicago, the results of the first study of an AI in women who did not have breast cancer were released. While sources like Medscape and the National Institutes of Health heralded the news about exemestane (Aromasin) as breast cancer "prevention," the June 4, 2011, *New York*

Times was more cautious, with a headline that read "Drug Can Reduce Breast Cancer Risk, Study Says."

And how were the results presented in the study? As relative risk reduction numbers, of course. All the press stories led with the news that women taking the drug in the trial reduced their risk of breast cancer by 65 percent.

The *New York Times* followed the 65 percent relative risk reduction numbers with the absolute risk reduction number, which is far different: about 0.9 percent. Imagine how the response to the story would have been different if it had led with this number instead.

According to the study, ninety-four women would need to be treated for three years with exemestane to prevent one case of breast cancer. That means that ninety-three women would be exposed to other effects that include bone pain, joint pain, and—noticeably missing from the list in the *New York Times*—osteoporosis. Most women on AIs for breast cancer develop osteoporosis, which means they get to take another drug to reduce the risk caused by the AI.

Know Your Numbers

In the Age of Health, we need to understand health numbers and their significance. Only with this information can we make intelligent decisions about treatment options and their risks. A great deal depends on understanding health numbers—maybe even your life.

June 13, 2011

Having a Voice, Communicating, and Somewhere in Between

I need to start this post with a disclaimer that may surprise you: I am not Christopher Hitchens. First of all, our politics are very different. More important for purposes of this post, Hitchens wrote a moving and erudite piece in *Vanity Fair* about the impact of losing his speaking voice to cancer (June 2011). It's worth reading.

ALS is robbing me of my speaking voice. For me, the onset of this damned progressive disease was with my speech: I started to have trouble enunciating words clearly. (That's how ALS starts in about one-third of people with the disease.) I'm now in a situation where it is most often very hard for me to project my voice beyond a whisper.

Followers of this blog know that some time ago I began using a voice amplifier ("There's That Person with . . . ," April 26, 2011). That doesn't help so much now. But, fortunately, there are other technologies.

Meet Kate

Many people with many different kinds of disabilities have known for a long time that technology makes continuing to be—and engage—in the world a possibility. For folks who have trouble talking, one form the technology takes is in programs that convert text to speech. I use a program called NeoKate, a free app for the iPad. I type in the text, tap on "done," and then Kate "says" what I typed.

Kate's English is pretty good, but she does have problems with some words, such as proper names and words that might have multiple pronunciations, like "read." So occasionally, after Kate attempts to pronounce what I've typed, I have to retype using phonetic spellings to get the words spoken correctly.

The program allows me to adjust Kate's speed (so I can make her sound like a native New Yorker if I want to), her pitch, and her volume. And if I want to save something I typed so I can have Kate speak it again later, there's a library where I can save files, with names I choose so I can find the files again later.

How Kate and I Behave in Company

In two-way conversations, using Kate to communicate slows things down a bit, since it always takes longer to type than to speak. It means there are longer pauses than there would be if two humans were talking to each other directly (without text-to-voice assistance). But it also means, at least so far in my experience, that people pay close attention to what Kate is saying for me, and it makes me listen more carefully to what's being said to me.

In conversations involving more than two people, Kate and I have a tougher time. You may have noticed that conversations often go off on tangents rather than following a straight line. You may also have noticed that sometimes people talk over each other—one person starts to say something before someone else finishes. When you add Kate to this mix, her part of the conversation can become quite disjointed. By the time I've finished typing a response to something someone said, the conversation may well have taken three other turns. When Kate says what I've typed, people have to stop to remember what the topic was that prompted the comment and get drawn back to a part of the conversation they thought was finished.

The delay has real impact on conversations. In a way, there is more continuity, in a disjointed way, than nontechnologically driven chats. Makes me think about those old ads from the brokerage firm E. F. Hutton: When Kate talks, people listen.

Can We Banter with Technology?

The m.o. for much conversation in my circles is banter: a statement is made, someone responds with a quip, and someone else answers the quip with another quip or statement or story. I love to banter, but my speaking ability won't let me do that anymore, and Kate's ability is limited by the time it takes for me to tell her what to say.

A friend of mine has suggested that we could even the conversational playing field by requiring everyone in the conversation to use Kate to communicate. That might be a little extreme, but we might all listen to each other better if we did something like this. On the other hand, we might all get so involved in typing our own stuff that we won't listen to other people's.

Given how ALS progresses, at some point (hopefully in the far distant future), it will become harder for me to type fast, or at all. Then, assuming (as I do) that I will continue to want to communicate, I will use technology that allows me to type by moving my eyes over characters on the computer screen. This process will inevitably be slower than the NeoKate method. The concept of "super slo-mo" will take on a whole new dimension. And the ability of other people to listen in this mode might be sorely tested.

So how I communicate in conversation with others—both how we talk and how well we listen—will be a growing issue for me. If it's an issue for me, it's an issue for everyone with whom I come in contact, and everyone else who is in the place of losing their speaking voices.

You may have noticed that this blog post is less about health policy—my usual topic—and more about social behavior. How we talk to each other affects how we hear each other, no matter what our limitations are or may become.

Think about it.

June 17, 2011

Walk for Your Health, but It Won't Help Anyone Else's, Much

A Little History on the "Walk for [Disease]" Thing

Back in 2000, I wrote a column for what was called then simply *The BCA Newsletter* titled "Exercise Your Mind" (March–April 2000). It was a critical look at what was then the Avon 3-Day Walk for Breast Cancer: how the money is raised, who gets to participate and who doesn't, the administrative costs of making the walks happen, and the lack of transparency about where the money raised for the cause actually ends up.

It is now more than a decade later and the criticism has been taken up by others: Samantha King wrote a book about it called *Pink Ribbons, Inc: Breast Cancer and the Politics of Philanthropy,* and a June 18, 2011, op-ed in the *New York Times* by Ted Gup was titled "The Weirdness of Walking to Raise Money." Yet the phenomenon of walking to raise money to cure diseases persists and grows.

Breast cancer is by far the biggest beneficiary of fund-raising walks: big ones are sponsored in multiple cities by the Susan G. Komen for the Cure Foundation (which took over the three-day walk from Avon), the Avon Foundation (philanthropic arm of the cosmetics company, which now hosts a two-day walk), the Revlon Foundation, and the American Cancer Society, to name a few. With all the walks going on, and all the money being raised with the promise of curing breast cancer, shouldn't breast cancer be cured by now?

How Fund-Raising Walks Work

All these walks have things in common:

- your family and friends asking you for money so they will be allowed to participate (there's always a minimum donation required)

- high administrative overhead, which means that of every dollar you give to support a walker, considerably less than a dollar goes to the cause you think you're supporting

- decisions made by the walk organizers, not the walkers, about where the money raised will be donated, which is often to places far from the community where the funds are raised

- an opportunity for people concerned about a particular disease to be together to share stories and support each other

From Overdone to Ridiculous

The walk thing has now gone far beyond breast cancer. You can walk "for" (Who is "for" diseases? Can we have a show of hands?) diabetes, birth defects, Alzheimer's disease, mental illness, epilepsy, hunger, and farm animals. The list goes on and on. You can even walk against abortion.

In what I think is the ultimate sad irony, there is a walk for ALS. You know, that disease that robs people like me who have it of the ability to walk.

Walk to Make a Real Difference

I still believe—and more so—what I thought in 2002 when I wrote that column for the BCA newsletter. Walk if you want to—it's good for your health. If you want to be sure your walking truly benefits people who are ill, walk to the nearest organization doing work you admire on the issue and lend a hand. You can even hand them a check if you're so inspired.

July 1, 2011

Thoughts on Dying and Living

L ast week, I had an e-mail from a friend wondering what I would say about Dudley Clendenin's op-ed in the Sunday, July 10 *New York Times* titled "The Good Short Life."

Seems that Mr. Clendenin and I have a few things in common: we're both from Baltimore (I moved away many years ago); more to the point, we both have ALS, the onset of which for both of us was with slurred speech, and we both think consciously about how we live our lives. In his op-ed, Mr. C wisely observes that we don't talk much in this country about how we die and that we all should be making conscious choices about that when the time comes.

For those of us with ALS and the people who love and care for us, it's impossible to imagine an outcome different from death. This reality diverges widely from my experience with breast cancer eighteen years ago. At that time, and for some time thereafter, I was intensely aware that there was no guarantee of tomorrow. I, along with my beloved partner, Susie, lived that reality for a while. Then the breast cancer diagnosis receded in time, and I got back to living for future things—like retirement, or that far-off trip to India.

Now, because of ALS, I am again faced with the stark reality that tomorrow is promised to no one. I'm also realizing both how hard it is to make sure my day-to-day life reflects this reality and, at the same time, how hard it is to be constantly reminded that this is where I am.

Because of ALS, there is almost no way I will ever get to live again as if I have a lot of time in front of me. And however much I want to take advantage of today, my ability to do that will become more and more limited as my illnesses progresses.

I don't want to die. But I will sooner than I would have thought less than a year ago. Mr. C, confronting the same reality, has decided to take control of his future by ending his life before his ALS becomes so advanced that his daughter will remember him horribly debilitated, or that he can't tie his bow tie or walk his dog.

In the meantime, he enjoyed a couple of wakes for himself that he got to attend. There's a celebration of me being planned for this September by folks here who know my work, and the one thing I'm insisting on is that it is *not* a funeral. There will be plenty of time for that—and for me to help plan it, for that matter, but I won't be there.

I'm pretty sure I will not want to end my life because I can't tie my shoes. There are always slip-ons, after all. But I also know that as my ALS progresses, I want to be able to make conscious choices about what I am willing to tolerate in terms of interventions and daily life. To do that, I need to keep focusing on what I value in life (love, music, words, time with people I care about, activities of the mind, pursuit of spiritual connection) and how much of what I value can be achieved or obtained when there is so much my body will not be able to do.

I want to cherish this time when I can do so much—and do as much as I can—even as I recognize how much more limited my abilities already are. And I want to keep my eyes wide open to what the future holds, realizing that I am essentially an optimist in how I approach life. This means that, even as my physical capabilities wane, I will look for and try to embrace the positive aspects in what remains available to me.

I think we respond to devastating health news from our essential beings. A fatal illness does not change who we are. Mr. C appears, from his column, to have an essential need to control the length of his ALS-compromised fate. By contrast, I think that I have an essential need to take the greatest advantage of the opportunities left in mine, though I recognize, as Mr. C does, that my need has implications for the lives of the people who care for me. Given who I essentially am, and who Mr. Clendenin appears to be from his column, I suspect he will die before I do, if that turns out to be in the control of either of us. I hope he dies as happily as he can, given that he has to go before he would want to if things were different. I hope the same for me when my time comes.

On a happier note, it seems another thing that Mr. C and I share is a love of Leonard Cohen. Like Mr. C, I hope for what Leonard Cohen writes about in his poem and song "Dance Me to the End of Love":

> Dance me to your beauty with a burning violin
> Dance me through the panic 'til I'm gathered safely in
> Lift me like an olive branch and be my homeward dove
> Dance me to the end of love

July 20, 2011

How Do You Spell Chutzpah?

K-o-m-e-n

Yiddish is a very expressive language, a blend of Hebrew and German used by Jews in Europe when they lived in shtetls. One of my favorite Yiddish words is *chutzpah*. The word has taken on some positive connotations, but I'm using it here in the sense of the Hebrew source word, where it means someone who has overstepped the boundaries of accepted behavior with no shame.

Chutzpah has the benefit of being both expressive and relatively easy to pronounce (unless you're Michele Bachmann). It is also a very apt description of the Susan G. Komen for the Cure Foundation's recent move to sponsor October as Breast Cancer Action Month.

The Longish Backstory

A little background might help illuminate why this move is so outrageous.

Back in the early 1980s, with the help of the pharmaceutical giant now called AstraZeneca, Komen (then called the Susan G. Komen Foundation—"for the cure" came later) became the dominant voice in Breast Cancer Awareness Month, formerly known as October. The idea was to encourage women to get mammograms by promising, at least initially, that early detection was a woman's best "prevention." When it was pointed out that once you had detected something, it was too late to prevent it, the message changed to guaranteeing that early detection was a woman's best "protection," though protection from what was never made clear.

Breast Cancer Awareness Month (BCAM) was largely sponsored by the pharmaceutical and mammography industries. Komen was— and is—closely tied to both. Thanks to the forces behind the BCAM effort, there was never any mention in the official BCAM materials of the possible environmental links to breast cancer. As a result, October came to be known in more progressive health circles as Breast Cancer Industry Month.

Breast Cancer Action (BCA), a national grassroots education and advocacy organization based in San Francisco, became a prominent voice working to recast October as Breast Cancer Industry Month. BCA was started in 1990 by women with metastatic breast cancer who knew that they were going to die and that the public knew little or less about breast cancer. They had questions and they wanted answers.

The messages offered by BCA for October moved far beyond mammography screening and the oversimplified messages associated with BCAM. They exposed the financial interests behind BCAM and urged an understanding of the complexity of "early detection" as well as acknowledgment of the environmental drivers of breast cancer, including radiation and pesticides (which AstraZeneca marketed at the time).

As the drum beat of breast cancer awareness reached deafening proportions, Breast Cancer Action encouraged people to look beyond awareness to what actions they could take by working together to stem the tide of breast cancer for everyone.

The Breast Cancer Trademark Business

Around the time that Breast Cancer Awareness Month came to the fore, Komen attempted unsuccessfully to trademark the pink ribbon, which was fast becoming the symbol of breast cancer.

More recently, Komen changed its name to the Susan G. Komen for the Cure Foundation and trademarked the phrase "for the cure." Komen then began suing other organizations that used "for the cure" in their name or fund-raising efforts, even those that had nothing to do with breast cancer. As of August 2010, Komen had more trademark applications pending with the U.S. Patent and Trade office (291) than Google (161).

Breast Cancer Action holds two trademarks: on its name and on the name of its Think Before You Pink® campaign.

Think Before You Pink® and Komen

One more bit of background information. When the marketing of breast cancer through the sale of products with pink ribbons on them began to grow, Breast Cancer Action initiated in 2002 its award-winning Think Before You Pink® campaign. The purpose of the campaign is to get people to think critically about how the money is raised and where the money goes.

The year that Think Before You Pink® was launched, a reporter from *PR Week* called asking why Breast Cancer Action had a campaign targeting Komen. The campaign targets cause marketing for breast cancer, not Komen. But the Komen Foundation has an interesting way of presenting—and apparently thinking of—itself as the only organization doing anything in the breast cancer world. It was clear then and as the campaign moved forward in succeeding years that Komen saw Think Before You Pink® as undermining its mission.

Now Komen Wants Action—*Breast Cancer Action?!?!*

It seems that Komen now agrees with BCA that there is enough awareness of breast cancer. After all, if you stop the first ten adults you see in the street and ask if they are aware there is a breast cancer problem in this country and elsewhere, anyone who says "no" must be living under a rock.

Komen wisely wants to move beyond awareness, but to what? They claim they want to move to "breast cancer action month." Has a familiar ring, right? It's often said that imitation is the sincerest form of flattery, but sometimes it's just a rip-off. Why would Komen, one of the biggest charities in the world, want to usurp the name of an organization that's been a thorn in their side for years? Let me think . . .

While it's conceivable that Komen just chose the words that they thought best suited their efforts, an organization that holds many trademarks and aggressively pursues them also has tons of lawyers at its disposal, and it should have crossed someone's mind to consider the possibility that an organization named Breast Cancer Action held a trademark that would affect their effort.

For Komen, action means getting a mammogram, buying product the sale of which supports Komen, or participating in a Race for the Cure or a three-day walk. If walking—or shopping—cured breast cancer, it would surely be cured by now.

Komen is entitled to its view of things, but not under the name of another—and very different—organization. If they want an even bigger empire, they should build it without stepping all over others in the field.

P.S. The American Cancer Society gets an honorary award for chutzpah, for its "official sponsor of birthdays" campaign. With mortality rates from many cancers increasing, and with the focus on five-year survival as a "cure," the cancer society is making a bold and unsubstantiated claim. Alcoholics Anonymous has far more basis for claiming to be the official sponsor of birthdays.

July 28, 2011

Drug Development and Access

Time to Act like Lives Depend on It

The Problem and the Incremental Solution

An op-ed in the Sunday *New York Times* in the past few weeks pointed out that important cancer drugs are being rationed by companies that have simply interrupted production (Ezekiel J. Emanuel, "Shortchanging Cancer Patients," *New York Times*, August 6, 2011). As a result, many cancer patients can't get the drugs they need.

Dr. Emanuel is an oncologist and a health policy wonk who was most recently an adviser in the Obama White House. In his article the good doctor details the current shortage of commonly used cancer drugs and what he sees as possible solutions to the problem. He clearly understands deeply the issues of cost reimbursement and the cost interaction between generics and patented drugs. He believes that the best way to get the missing drugs back on the market is to make generics of the drugs that are in short supply more profitable.

Capitalism and Health Care: Not a Good Mix

The article got me thinking once more about whether capitalism and health care are concepts that make any sense together, and about how cancer and ALS are different yet the same.

In his op-ed, Dr. Emanuel says, "You don't have to be a cynical capitalist to see that the long-term solution is to make the production of generic cancer drugs more profitable."

I see the situation differently: you don't have to be a raging

191

socialist to see that the solution to the drug access and cost problem is to nationalize the pharmaceutical industry. We can pass laws until the cows come home to try to get pharmaceutical companies to behave in ways that will not harm patients while keeping their profits intact. But the goal of companies that make drugs is to make money, and that goal will always trump the needs of patients when the two conflict. Sadly, you can bet your life on it.

As long as we insist that health care must provide a profit for the drug companies and that this profit must not be subject to regulation, our health will be shortchanged.

Meanwhile, the shortage of cancer drugs is dire and getting worse as patients await the arrival of prescribed medicines so they can start or continue the treatment that may extend or improve their lives.

Cancer and ALS: Different Diseases, Similar Issues

The cancer treatment situation is terrible. Equally, but differently, bad is the situation with ALS, where there is only one drug approved to treat the disease. That drug is Rilutek (riluzole). If it works—and it doesn't work for everyone—it delays progression of the disease for up to nine months. It does nothing to make you feel or function better and nothing to extend your life.

The absence of ALS drugs is in part the result of the fact that the market is so small: because, relative to cancer and many other diseases, so few people have ALS. That means there is not as much profit to be made from ALS drugs. But that doesn't mean that the research resources are so limited that we can address only the diseases for which drugs can be profitably made. It simply means that there's not enough potential profit in ALS drugs or drugs to treat other relatively untreatable diseases (like pancreatic or head and neck cancers, to name just a few) to make the research attractive to private companies.

Potential profit will continue to be an incentive to develop drugs for diseases that are relatively widespread. What we need are incentives to push the research also in the direction of, if you will, "less profitable" diseases that need treatments. What would happen if national policy *required* drug development for diseases that are always or nearly always fatal, and for which there are very few if any good treatment options? I'm sure there are many people who would take issue with this standard, but maybe we should have the conversation and think about whether and how it might work.

In my opinion, it's time to get away from niggling around the edges of how to make capitalism and drug development (or health care in general) work together. Maybe it's time to put patients' needs first. Isn't that a nifty idea?

August 18, 2011

Science by Press Release—
Not Good News for Patients

It May Look Like News

If you have ALS, or know someone who does, you were probably inundated with e-mails from well-meaning and loving friends earlier this week with the news of a "breakthrough" in ALS research. I first saw the news in the press release issued by Northwestern University, the institution that sponsored the research. The headlines of many of the stories that resulted from that press release read "Major ALS Breakthrough: Researchers Discover Common Cause of All Forms of ALS." Don't go running to the pharmacy for the new treatment for ALS. It's not here yet. It's not even close.

As a longtime health activist, I am more than a little bit familiar with what I have come to call "science by press release." A research institution finds something interesting, they widely distribute a press release putting the best possible spin on it, and the media outlets run with the story. Try a Google search of the phrase "ALS breakthrough" and see how many hits you get.

What Does It Mean for Patients?

The first question to ask when you see a story about a medical breakthrough is, "What does this mean for patients today?" In the case of this ALS story, nada. What has been found is a protein called Ubiquilin 2 that occurs in spinal and brain system cells. It's supposed to repair or dispose of other proteins as they become damaged. The researchers discovered a breakdown of this function in ALS patients.

This may prove to be good news, especially if it is confirmed by other research and drugs can be developed to address the damaged protein. But we're a long way from that day, and many things could happen that keep researchers from getting to it. For example, it may turn out that some other protein or proteins have to be controlled to make sure that Ubiquilin 2 functions properly. The unknown territory is vast.

Key Words to Look For

There are key words to watch for in the science-by-press-release world. Among them are *breakthrough*, *advance*, and *may*, *might*, or *could lead to*. When you see these words in a story about a medical breakthrough, listen carefully for what's being reported. Far more often than not, the story is about something that worked in the lab but hasn't been tried yet in patients, or about a study of a very small number of patients.

Those of us living with illness, and the people who love and care about us, need hope. But we don't need research masquerading as news that will affect our chances of surviving. As one scientist interviewed on the ALS story said, "You need to understand at the cellular level what is going wrong. Then you can begin to design drugs." Call me when you get there.

Dreaming

When I was the executive director of Breast Cancer Action, I often wished that a PhD candidate would review all the news stories in the past decade about medical breakthroughs in breast cancer and figure out which ones in fact resulted in improving outcomes for patients. I would love to read that dissertation.

What You Can Do

Next time you see a medical "breakthrough" story, think about contacting the media outlet and telling (or just asking) them what their story means to patients today, especially if it may be, might be, or probably is nothing.

August 26, 2011

Health Activism—
Not for the Faint of Heart

I have been a health activist since 1994. Having spent a long time in the cancer field, it seems that now I am destined to become an ALS activist. I just can't seem to help myself.

Wearing One Hat

I think a lot about what it means to be a health activist and how that differs from being an advocate. When I was a member of the California Breast Cancer Research Council, I would show up at meetings and claim my name card for the conference table. On it would be printed my name, my organization, and the word *advocate*. That title was there because the legislation that created the program required that a certain number of council representatives be "advocates."

My experience in breast cancer taught me that many, if not most, people who called themselves advocates had no clear sense of what they were advocating for. Many of them represented two—and often more—different organizations with different missions and objectives, and they would tout the position of whichever organization suited their purposes at the moment. Others went from one organization to another until they found a place where they could claim their views as those of the group.

In my lexicon, an *activist* is someone who is clear about her/his goals and strategic about achieving them. S/he cannot be bought—no amount of money or privileges will change her commitment to her goals.

Clear Goals

In breast cancer, there are many goals that require activism, for example, better detection devices, better treatments, better access to detection and treatment for everyone, uniting and refocusing the research agenda, and fighting breast cancer "fatigue" brought on by pink ribbon marketing. While some activists take on more than one of these issues at a time, all will require a lot of effort by a lot of people.

In ALS, the issues seem by contrast much easier to list. They are, however, no easier to achieve. In fact, I can think of only two at the moment (though I'm relatively speaking new to ALS, so the list may grow): better treatments and access for everyone affected to the kind of care that will improve the quality of their lives.

Challenges for ALS Activists

One of the differences between breast cancer activism and ALS activism is that many people survive breast cancer for a long time, so many people have time and energy to get involved. With ALS, while some people live a long time, the disease is always fatal and always robs people of some physical abilities. It's harder to be an engaged activist. So we do what we can.

Beyond Self-Interest

Regardless of the disease at issue, a health activist is also someone for whom her goals, while they might benefit her personally once they are achieved, are aimed at affecting people she doesn't even know. The goals are about more than self-interest: they are about changing systems so that many people who now suffer will benefit. More often than not, those goals and objectives are bigger than can be achieved in one lifetime, and activists know that their efforts are possible because of previous work done by others. They also know that if they do their job right, others will come after them to advance the work.

Taking the Heat and Keeping an Open Mind

Health activists have to be tough. Because they publicly take princi-
pled positions, there are always people who disagree with them and
say so, sometimes in not-so-nice terms. If an activist caves because her
positions have been criticized, she's not really an activist.

I learned this lesson many times in my breast cancer work.
When I criticized raising money by putting pink ribbons on products to promote sales, many people got angry, wondering how anyone
could criticize money being raised for breast cancer. When I argued
that the drug Avastin should not be sold for treatment of breast cancer, I was accused of sentencing women to an early death. And when
I endorsed the mammography screening guidelines that would end
routine screening of women between ages forty and forty-nine, I was
told I would have blood on my hands.

ALS is not as prominent as breast cancer. But when I recently
posted my blog titled "Science by Press Release—Not Good News for
Patients" to a site for ALS patients, there were a lot of people who
disagreed with me, saying I was depriving them of hope. I'm used
to this. If you're an activist who can't get used to it, you might want to
find another line of work.

This doesn't mean that activists never change their positions, but
it does mean that those changes are the result of changed conditions
or developments that compel a shift in position because the old positions don't make sense anymore.

Doing the Work, Getting the Rewards

Activists want to make the world better for people. They are committed, tough, and they are not afraid to speak their minds. Many are
willing to learn the nitty-gritty of the issues with which they are dealing so that they can engage in intelligent conversations with people
who have power on those issues.

Being an activist is not for the faint of heart. But the rewards are
often great. You meet great people, you learn a great deal, and sometimes, just sometimes, you make a difference in the world.

September 8, 2011

Pink Ribbons and Lou Gehrig

Time to Bury Useless Symbols

People who have known me a while know that I'm no fan of pink ribbons as a symbol for breast cancer. I have the same feeling about baseball slugger Lou Gehrig as a symbol for ALS. It's time to let go of symbols that have become useless or, worse, misleading.

A Brief History of Breast Cancer's Pink Ribbon

The first breast cancer ribbon was not pink.

It was salmon colored. It was created by a woman named Charlotte Haley, who had seen a lot of her family struggle with breast cancer. Charlotte wanted to see more done to address the breast cancer epidemic. Inspired by the AIDS ribbon, she created salmon-colored ribbons out of cloth, put five of them on a postcard encouraging people to contact their elected representatives, and sold the postcards for five bucks each so she could make more.

Estée Lauder, the cosmetics company, and *Self* magazine, a women's publication, quickly recognized the profit-making possibilities of the ribbon. They approached Charlotte, claiming that they cared deeply about women and wanted to make her ribbon the international symbol of breast cancer. Charlotte thought that was more about the companies' bottom lines than about women's lives and refused to partner with them.

The companies were advised by their lawyers that they could use a ribbon; they should just find another color. So the companies asked focus groups of women to identify the color or colors that were most reassuring, nonthreatening, and comforting—everything a breast cancer diagnosis is *not*. The color they came up with was pink.

The Komen Foundation (now called the Susan G. Komen for the Cure Foundation) tried to trademark the pink ribbon. When that failed, everyone and their grandmother starting using it to symbolize breast cancer. Briefly put, because anyone can use the pink ribbon, everyone does, from marketers of products to huge organizations. The pink ribbon has made it possible for breast cancer to become the poster child of cause marketing by companies trying to improve their sales by linking their products to the breast cancer cause. Some people and companies merely sell ribbons (made of everything from cloth to platinum and diamonds) and keep all the revenues; others use it to promote sales of other products (everything from toilet paper, to cars, to guns) by promising to donate a "portion" of the proceeds to breast cancer research. Sometimes the ribbons are placed on products that are bad for our health.

How Many Things Can a Pink Ribbon Cover Up?

Billions of dollars have been raised in the name of breast cancer research. We don't know how much of that money actually goes to research. We don't know what kinds of research are funded with that money. And the research funders often tout how much they have spent without ever reporting whether the research has benefited women's lives. What we do know is that the epidemic rages on, the incidence of breast cancer continues to increase, and the death rate does not decline.

When you ask most people what they know about breast cancer, if they can say anything, they will say something about the importance of mammograms. But there is so much more to breast cancer. To name just a few things that the pink ribbon doesn't represent: the limits of early detection, the ineffectiveness of current treatments to keep women with metastatic breast cancer from dying, the environmental triggers of the disease (only at most 10 percent of breast cancer is caused by an inherited genetic mutation), and the racial inequities in both the incidence and mortality rate from breast cancer.

Many of these issues are illuminated in the new documentary from the National Film Board of Canada, *Pink Ribbons, Inc.*, by director Léa Pool and producer Ravida Din.[1] The film was inspired by a book of the same title by Samantha King.[2] The film is now being shown at film festivals outside the United States. It should be in theaters here by February 2012.

If we're going to focus on what needs to happen to end the scourge of breast cancer, we need to find a new symbol, one that actually conveys the impact of the disease on people's lives and that doesn't lend itself so readily to corporate exploitation or to covering up the realities of breast cancer.

Maybe if we put our heads together we can come up with a new symbol. Ideas?

Lou Gehrig: May He Rest in Peace?

Lou Gehrig died of ALS in 1941 at the age of thirty-seven. Many people who think they have never heard of ALS have heard of Lou Gehrig's disease, the "popular" name for this devastating illness. By now, more people probably know Gehrig for his illness than for his baseball prowess.

Gehrig died more than seventy years ago. Since he died, many more people, some of them quite well known, have died of ALS. Yet in nearly every story about ALS, Gehrig's name appears, often with a picture of the baseball player standing hale and hearty with a baseball bat in his hand. He doesn't look sick, let alone devastated by the physical ravages of ALS.

Is it any wonder that the public doesn't understand what ALS is when the symbol they see is so unrelated to the realities of the disease? Wouldn't a better symbol convey the real-life circumstances of twenty-first-century people with ALS? Just because "Lou Gehrig" is easier to say than amyotrophic lateral sclerosis doesn't mean that Lou Gehrig is a good symbol for the disease today.

Good Symbols for a Change

For people to be motivated to care about and work to change either breast cancer or ALS, they need to understand what these illnesses are and how they affect people today. Appropriate symbols can help convey that understanding. Let's find and use symbols that at least hint at the realities so that people might—just might—be motivated to change them.

September 18, 2011

Notes

1. *Pink Ribbons, Inc.*, directed by Léa Pool (New York: First Run Features, 2011), DVD.

2. Samantha King, *Pink Ribbons, Inc.: Breast Cancer and the Politics of Philanthropy* (Minneapolis: University of Minnesota Press, 2008).

Mi Shebeirach

Thoughts on Illness and Blessing

This long essay was prompted by my thoughts about the Jewish New Year, the Jewish Day of Atonement, and the prayer that Jews say for healing. Grab a cup of your favorite hot beverage, and settle in. As always, feel free to share. And L'Shana Tova (Happy New Year).

At 2011 Yom Kippur services (Jewish services for the Day of Atonement), with the help of my partner, Susie Lampert, I delivered the following teaching using a text-to-speech program that allows me to express my thoughts in spoken words even though my ability to speak is quite compromised. The program is called NeoKate. It's a free app for the iPad.

Last year at this time, I was on the verge of turning fifty-nine. Yesterday, I turned sixty. God willing, next year I will turn sixty-one. But the medical unknown I faced last year, that I told you about then on the afternoon of Rosh Hashanah, has turned into a dreaded disease: ALS. There is no cure. There aren't even any good treatments. So, barring the end of the world as I know it, or a medical miracle, I know how I will die and that my life will be shorter and my living far more compromised than I would have ever thought or wished it to be.

As my ALS progresses, I want to be able to make conscious choices about what I am willing to tolerate in terms of interventions and daily life. To do that, I need to keep focusing on what I value in life—love, music, words, time with people I care about, activities of the mind, pursuit of spiritual connection—and how much of what I value can be achieved or obtained when there is so much my body will not be able to do.

And I want to keep my eyes wide open to what the future holds, realizing that I am essentially an optimist in how I approach life. I think we respond to devastating health news from our essential beings. A fatal illness does not change who we are. For me this means that, even as my physical capabilities wane, I will look for and try to embrace the positive aspects in what remains available to me.

Illness confronts us with some of the greatest uncertainties we ever face. In my case—and really for all of us—the uncertainty is not about what the future holds, but how it will unfold. How do we embrace illness, if that is our reality, without welcoming it? How do we continue to do what matters to us as long as we can? How do we find comfort in the support of friends and the love of God? What role does God play in a devastating illness and in healing?

These issues are particularly poignant during the Days of Awe, and especially at Yom Kippur. As my Rabbi, Margaret Holub, reminded me, one important part of the Yom Kippur ritual is rehearsing our own deaths as we fast, repent, dress in the white of a shroud, and engage in the recitation of the culminating Shema (the central prayer of the Jewish faith) in the divine presence that closes the Day of Atonement.

But the prayer we say for healing—the Mi Shebeirach—is said whenever the Torah (the first five books of the Old Testament) is read and at many other times as well. Healing is by no means limited to Yom Kippur. And there are quite a few translations of the prayer, which originated, interestingly enough, as a prayer for rain in a time of drought. I'm partial to Debbie Friedman's version, which can be stated briefly as:

> May the source of strength,
> Who blessed the ones before us,
> Help us find the courage
> To make our lives a blessing

And let us say, Amen
Bless those in need of healing with r'fuah sh'leimah
The renewal of body, the renewal of spirit
And let us say, Amen

The new facts of my life also brought back to me the soliloquy from *Hamlet* that was central to the teaching on uncertainty that I did here last year on Rosh Hashanah. Most people know the part of this speech that starts "To be, or not to be," but there are other words that speak to me:

But that the dread of something after death,
The undiscover'd country from whose bourn
No traveller returns, puzzles the will,
And makes us rather bear those ills we have
Than fly to others that we know not of?
Thus conscience does make cowards of us all,
And thus the native hue of resolution
Is sicklied o'er with the pale cast of thought,
And enterprises of great pitch and moment
With this regard their currents turn awry,
And lose the name of action.

The Friedman translation of the Mi Shebeirach prayer is really not so far removed from *Hamlet*. I think asking for the courage to make our lives a blessing has a lot in common with avoiding the fear that puzzles the will and makes us lose the name of action.

That *Hamlet* quotation also has things in common, I think, with comments Rabbi Margaret made at the start of Rosh Hashanah (the Jewish New Year) this year about what it would be like to live conscious of all the terror and awe that are part of the world that God created. Nothing like an always-fatal disease to remind me that this is actually where I now live all the time. How do we face this reality and keep moving forward?

One aspect of my answer to this question is nicely expressed in one of the meditations at the beginning of our High Holy Day prayer book:

> Awe is an intuition for the creaturely dignity of all things and
> their preciousness to God; a realization that things not only are
> what they are but also stand, however remotely, for something
> absolute. Awe is a sense for the transcendent, for the reference
> everywhere to God, who is beyond all things. Awe enables us
> to perceive in the world intimations of the divine, to sense in
> small things the beginning of infinite significance, to sense the
> ultimate in the common and the simple; to feel in the rush of
> the passing the stillness of the eternal.

One way for me to keep the terror in perspective is to focus on the places where God's awe is manifest. As I'm less able to get around, I notice a lot of things through the front window of our house: hummingbirds, the clouds in the sky, the quality of the light. In the right frame of mind, I draw from these things the sense of the transcendent, of the reference everywhere to God. They enable me to sense in small things the beginning of infinite significance.

Within this framework of awe and terror, I keep moving forward—which is another way of not losing the name of action, of trying to make my life a blessing—I am determined to do what I can, while I can, and to adapt to do things differently as I lose function. I'm an activist by nature or nurture or experience. As I lose mobility, I have acquired a cane and walker to help me get around on foot. I use eating utensils with fat handles, which are easier for me to grip than regular utensils. Since I can't talk very well, I write a blog that keeps me engaged in the world and interacting with people who care about the things I care and write about, and I speak with the help of technology. I spend time with my beloved partner, Susie. I travel as I can to places I need or want to be.

And over the course of the past year, as I have worked to face my reality with my eyes open and without losing the name of action, I have found myself looking in many places for how to do that. One such place is my Jewish heritage. With Rabbi Margaret's help, I have taken up weekly Torah study with a dear friend (in English; I can't read Hebrew). I fulfilled a goal that had long been in my mind of taking a Hebrew name, and I decided to do that before I learned that some Jews change their Hebrew names when they are seriously ill to try to fool the angel of death. As part of the process of taking a Hebrew name, I immersed in a Mikvah (a Jewish ritual bath) for the first time. I now meet regularly with a rabbi from the Jewish Healing Center in San Francisco.

As I read Torah, I find things that help me maintain perspective on healing and faith. In the part of Genesis called Mikeitz, the following commentary appears in the *Etz Hayim* version of the Torah: "One of the lessons of the Joseph story . . . is that life is cyclical. Good years are followed by lean years, adversity is followed by success, rejection yields connection, winter gives way to spring and summer, only to return again. What can be learned from this *parashah* is to prepare ourselves in the good days, days in which holiness is revealed, to set the light in our hearts, to be there in times when holiness seems far off." The author of *S'fat Emet* answers his own question: "We must store up resources of faith, even as the Egyptians stored grain, to nourish us spiritually when events turn against us."

From Rabbi Eric Weiss of the Jewish Healing Center I have learned to return, either physically or in my mind, to the places in nature that feed my soul without being nostalgic for how I used to be in those places. Instead, I see the beauty in these places in the way I can now, given my physical limitations.

I also spend time with friends, though this has posed a greater challenge for me in some ways. My energy is not what it was, and I need to be careful not to overdo either physically or emotionally. But there is the mitzvah (good deed) of visiting the sick, called *bikkur holim*. I have struggled with this directive, as the object of the mitzvah. Finally, I concluded that the directive about the mitzvah is directed at the visitor, not the person who is ill. While it is a mitzvah to visit the sick, that does not require the person who is ill to see everyone who is trying to fulfill it. I have it on good authority from the Shulcan Aruch that the rule is that if you go to visit a sick person who is not up to seeing you, you should stay in the hall and sweep the floor. My friends have been mostly understanding and are kind enough to metaphorically sweep the hall floor from time to time.

I have also learned that support of my community—people I know and even people I don't—is enormously important to my spiritual healing. When people tell me they have said the Mi Shebeirach for me, it touches me and helps me. According to the *Etz Hayim* Torah commentary, we say this prayer for two reasons: to ask for God's help in healing those who are ill and to notify the community who is ill and in need of the support of the community.

When we said this prayer last week at Rosh Hashanah services in Mendocino, California, the number of names recited as in need of healing was startling to me. The number of calls on the community (and most communities, I imagine) for acts of support and loving kindness, which I experience whenever I am with the Jewish community in Mendocino, may seem daunting. But as one commentator put it, the prayer seems to act less as a wish for literal fulfillment of a petition and more as means to set one's heart in the right direction. Invoking God's blessing can be a boon, regardless of what God does or does not do—because it enables the person who is ill to be joined in her suffering by divine presence.

When Rabbi Weiss blesses me at the end of our monthly sessions, I feel that presence. When this congregation says the Mi Shebeirach, I feel it, too.

In Debbie Friedman's version of the Mi Shebeirach, the verses end with the phrase "and let us say, Amen." I believe that when we call together for healing and spiritual connection, it helps those of us who are ill. All of us are deeply grateful.

And let us say, "Amen."

October 10, 2011

Is October over Yet?

October is often a beautiful fall month. It's also my birthday month. But I learned early in my tenure at Breast Cancer Action to dread the month because everything turned pink. I had hoped that when I stepped down from my job, I could get back to having October just be a month. But once a breast cancer activist, always one, I guess. So I still feel inundated in October.

Pinktober

This month has so far been no exception. It's hard to decide what the worst offender was among the things that turned pink this month. Was it the garbage truck for the cure in New York City? Was it the oil rig painted pink? Was it the Lord & Taylor Pink Carpet of Beauty? Was it American Airlines (the only airline currently losing money) Fly for the Cure effort? Or was the winner the pink cleats on those NFL football players as they pummeled each other on a recent Sunday? Or maybe it was the Komen for the Cure Foundation's Promise Me perfume, laced with a lot of ingredients that are known to increase the risk of cancer.

Maybe you have a favorite in the "how low can we go with pink" contest. If you do, send it to Breast Cancer Action so it can be used in the organization's Think Before You Pink® campaign.

A Ray of Sanity from the *New York Times*? Sadly Not

I don't read the Sunday *New York Times* in October or any other month. I won't spend the kind of time it requires to read it carefully. I figure that if there's an important article in it, a friend will tell me about it or I'll stumble on it in the iPad *New York Times* app. But probably because of my background, I did quickly find an article published by the *Times* on October 15 that gave me a little hope that we would finally have an in-depth investigative report about the pinking of America. After all, the new (and first female) executive editor of the paper says she is dedicated to more investigative reporting.

Titled "Welcome, Fans, to the Pinking of America," the article by Natasha Singer appeared, appropriately enough, as the lead story in the paper's business section. So far, so good. And early on there are acknowledgments that not everyone likes the pinking of everything. But it becomes quickly clear that the article is about how successful the Komen Foundation has been in making breast cancer into a multibillion dollar marketing opportunity to support mammography screening and breast cancer education, and not about how this effort has left most of the public completely in the dark about the realities of breast cancer.

The article quotes Nancy Brinker, the founder of Komen, as follows: "It's a democratization of a disease. It's drilling down into the deepest pockets of America." So this is what democracy means, getting money out of anyone you can find? Funny, I thought it meant people participating in the political process by which decisions that affect their lives are made. How did we get to this?

I blame the Komen Foundation, the leading but not the only beneficiary of products sold with pink ribbons on them. It is Komen that has, in the article's words, "rebranded an entire disease by putting an upbeat spin on fighting it." And it's done that by marketing and by drilling into the buying public messages that are wrongheaded in the extreme. Those messages range from how much progress has been made in breast cancer to how mammograms are all anyone needs to know about breast cancer.

One thing that the *New York Times* article makes clear is that, while consumers are encouraged to buy products to support breast cancer research, Komen spends twice as much on education as it does on research. So if you think that by buying pink you're funding research, think again.

I won't attempt to summarize the rest of the *New York Times* article, since it is mostly a promotion of Komen's approach. While it mentions that Komen's message may oversimplify breast cancer issues, it hardly says why or how.

Words from Komen: Same Song, Different Verse

While Pinktober was raging and the buying opportunities mounted, I was the unhappy recipient of a fund-raising letter from Komen. Seems the millions that the foundation raises from corporate partnerships aren't enough, so they do a lot of direct mail. The letter contains the following statements:

- Komen funds "research dedicated to conquering breast cancer at every stage—from the causes to the cures."
- "Our single-minded focus [is] on finding the cures."
- "We're working 24/7 to find the cures for breast cancer."
- "Imagine life without breast cancer."

Most of the letter focuses on how much Komen funding has accomplished and how Komen is going to fund the cures for breast cancer if I write a big check (not). But what does it mean to "imagine life without breast cancer"? I don't know how I can do that with so few resources devoted to finding and eradicating the causes of the disease. And while the letter mentions in passing that Komen funds this kind of research, I know for a fact that it is a very small part of the foundation's portfolio and that they ignore many of the findings that come from that research. The foundation's information about environmental links to breast cancer is flat-out wrong in a lot of places.

At the invitation of someone associated with an organization called the Breast Cancer Sisterhood, Komen agreed to respond on a blog hosted by the Sisterhood to questions and criticisms raised by others in the breast cancer "community."[1] The person who wrote on behalf of Komen is the "Director of Marketing and Communications."

Though there was supposed to be a give-and-take with the Komen representative, she (the Komen rep) posted one message defending Komen and failed to answer many questions. As far as I can tell she hasn't responded to subsequent comments. So much for dialogue.

And Komen is not alone in claiming the ground of funding all the progress in breast cancer.

The Breast Cancer Research Foundation (BCRF) took out a couple of full-page ads in the *New York Times* to tell people how so much of the progress in breast cancer it has funded. It reads a lot like Komen's claims. Of particular note to me is that much of the funding for BCRF comes from not just pink products but directly from the Estée Lauder Companies. They make cosmetics and they founded BCRF, which is committed to "prevention and a cure in our lifetime." The first part will be particularly tricky so long as Estée Lauder refuses to sign the *Compact for Safe Cosmetics* and continues to use toxins in their products.[2] Hypocrisy? You betcha.

Seems all the big players use Pinktober to cover up one thing or another about breast cancer.

A Word about Mammograms

Since Komen thinks everyone should get a mammogram, and that's all they talk about in October, a couple of things of note on this topic.

Just as the month was drawing to a close, a new study was issued that shows that mammograms result in a great deal of overtreatment and actually only help at most 13 percent of women whose breast cancer is found by mammogram (that's about 18,000 women per year of the 138,000 diagnosed by mammograms). I could go into a long explanation about why this is true, but Breast Cancer Action has already done a pretty good job of explaining it. Take a look at the organization's policy on *Screening and Early Detection*, particularly the section starting on page three about the biological complexity of breast cancer and its impact on early detection.[3] Maybe if the folks at Komen read it they would learn something.

Komen, of course, is not alone in encouraging mammograms even when they are not called for. There's an organization called Rethink Breast Cancer that is using soft porn to encourage women to get screened. They've even made this message into a smart phone app (http://www.youtube.com/watch?v=VsyE2rCW710). Is it any wonder that I want October to end, and soon?

October 29, 2011

Notes

1. This is the blog hosted by the Sisterhood: http://breastcancersister hood.com/brendas-blog/.

2. For more on the compact, see the Campaign for Safe Cosmetics Web site at http://safecosmetics.org/article.php?list=type&type=32.

3. See http://bcaction.org/wp-content/uploads/2011/01/BCA-Screen ing-Policy-Final-2010.pdf. For BCAction's updated and current policies on screening and other issues, see www.bcaction.org.

Labyrinth

Susie and I had a fabulous day and a half in the redwoods of southern Humboldt County. We stayed in Garberville and walked on the accessible paths of Humboldt Redwoods State Park. Since these big, magnificent trees are my home away from home, it was a perfect couple of days in an exquisite place with the love of my life. What could be hard about that?

I guess what could be hard is the reaction that some of you might have had to my previous journal post updating my health situation. I know it's a lot to absorb (imagine how I feel about that ☺—both that news and the notion that I'm becoming physically very different from the person a lot of you have known. I understand that using Caring Bridge to stay connected with folks is one [medium] with which different people will have varying levels of comfort. I also know that you love me and that each of you has to figure out how to be with me, either virtually or in person, as my health changes.

If it's not possible for you to spend time with me in person, I would love it if you would pray for me (or think good thoughts, if you're not a person who prays), send photos of beautiful places in nature that you love, toast me when you're out for drinks, or just think of me from time to time. It helps me spiritually. Truly it does.

My spiritual self also got a boost today. My walker and I "took a spin" with my dear friend Margie on the outdoor labyrinth at Grace Cathedral. My friendship with Margie grew up on labyrinth walks, and it was wonderful to have that experience again. As I walked the intricate path through the circle, I thought about life, love, laughter, and loss and how they are one big circle. Thanks to you all, I still have all of them.

Love, Barbara

December 8, 2011

IOM Report on Breast Cancer and the Environment

What Komen's One Million Dollars Bought

E arly this month the Institute of Medicine (IOM), an arm of the National Academy of Sciences, released a report on environmental links to breast cancer. The IOM describes itself as "an independent, nonprofit organization that works outside of government to provide unbiased and authoritative advice to decision makers and the public."[1] In this case, the IOM was given $1 million by the Susan G. Komen for the Cure Foundation (Komen), which asked the IOM to "review the current evidence on breast cancer and the environment, consider gene-environment interactions, review the research challenges, explore evidence-based actions that women might take to reduce their risk, and recommend directions for future research."

By defining *environment* broadly to include lifestyle factors, the IOM report covers both involuntary exposures (those that require policy changes to control) and voluntary exposures (such as smoking and diet, including alcohol consumption) and focuses its risk reduction recommendations on the latter. (The IOM "Opportunities for Actions" document is all about how women need to protect themselves.)[2] These recommendations will only reinforce the inclination of women to blame themselves when they get breast cancer.

The results of the report are hardly either surprising or overwhelming. In fact, the report repeats what has been known for more than a decade. The IOM summarizes its conclusions this way: "Overall, the IOM finds that major advances have been made in understanding breast cancer and its risk factors, but more needs to be learned about its causes and how to prevent it. The report urges a life-course approach to studying breast cancer because new information suggests that women and girls might be more susceptible to some risk factors during certain life stages."

The life-course approach has been advocated for a long time. The National Institutes of Health Breast Cancer and the Environment Research Centers have been funding this kind of research since 2003 (http://www.bcerc.org/home.htm). So the IOM report does not break new ground. Worse, it is silent on policy changes required to reduce involuntary exposures to toxins that may be contributing to the skyrocketing rates of breast and other cancers.

We should not be surprised. Here's why.

A Little Background

When I was executive director at Breast Cancer Action, Komen spent half a million dollars for a review of all the published scientific information on environmental links to breast cancer. That review, conducted by the Silent Spring Institute, was published in June 2007 in the American Cancer Society's journal *Cancer*. For people concerned about the issue of environmental links to breast cancer, it was a watershed moment. The study was widely reported and applauded. Many researchers took to heart the ideas presented about how to approach more studies in the field.

In December 2007—the year of the Silent Spring study—I met with the then-CEO of Komen, Hala Moddelmog, and the organization's then-policy director, Diane Balma. (Moddelmog left Komen to become president of Arby's Restaurant Group. Enough said.) My intention was to thank them for funding the report and to explore ways that Komen and Breast Cancer Action might work together to advance its recommendations.

I started the conversation by thanking the Komen reps for funding the Silent Spring study. Ms. Moddelmog responded by asking me if anyone was finding it useful. It was clear to me from the question that Komen had funded the study but not followed its publication or use. How sad.

The reason that Komen has been so reluctant to look at chemical exposures is not hard to discern. Komen's corporate partnerships are well known to most people in the breast cancer world. Komen is basically a wholly owned subsidiary of corporate America. But not many people have thought about how those connections—to companies like Ford Motor Company, for example—inhibit what research Komen might be willing to do on toxins linked to breast cancer that come out of the tailpipes of cars. A very few people have even noticed that Komen is marketing a perfume called Promise Me that contains known or probable carcinogens (http://bcaction.org/take-action/raise-a-stink/).

The Radiation Connection

There are very few things that we can say with certainty cause breast cancer. One of those things is *ionizing radiation* (http://www.silent spring.org/risk-factors-breast-cancer). Not that everyone exposed will get breast cancer, but the risk goes up with exposure, and we know the biological mechanism of the process.

While the IOM report urges individuals to reduce their exposure to medical radiation, it says nothing about policy changes to reduce everyone's exposure to this risk, including rethinking our approach to routine breast cancer screening using mammography, which is radiation based.

Komen is the biggest promoter of more and more mammography. This fact, and the fact that Komen funded the IOM report, may explain why there is no recommendation in the report for the medical community to monitor and limit radiation exposures.

Which brings me back to my meeting with Moddelmog and Balma. When I suggested in 2007 that Komen and Breast Cancer Action might work together to encourage women to track and limit their exposure to ionizing radiation, I was immediately told that was a nonstarter, because doing so would discourage women from getting mammograms.

The irony here is that all three of us in the conversation had had breast cancer, all three had had regular mammograms, and *in none of our cases* was the breast cancer found by mammogram.

So whether it's radiation or toxic chemicals, Komen is boxed in by its positions and partnerships. And that means that no report funded by Komen will ever recommend actions that challenge the profitability of its corporate partners or suggest that the organization rethink its core message about mammograms. That also means that as long as Komen dominates the conversation about breast cancer, the rest of us are pretty much screwed.

Independent Research? Not by a Long Shot

With that background, consider how the IOM is constrained when it gets funding for its research from an organization like Komen. When Komen defines the research question as broadly as it did, the research results are destined to look as they do: like a repeat of all we already know.

Where Do We Go from Here?

Komen, having purchased with $1 million just the kind of advice it wanted, says it will now invest in the kind of research called for by the IOM report. But because the report includes so many things as "environmental," it will be entirely possible for Komen to invest in research of anything but toxic chemicals.

Already Komen has spent $1.5 million on research into what the research agenda should be. The IOM report gives Komen just the cover it wanted to avoid looking at involuntary chemical exposures as a culprit in the breast cancer epidemic.

It's time for a change. E-mail Liz Thompson, CEO of Komen: tell her you want Komen to invest in research on chemicals that may be linked to breast cancer.

And contact the Institute of Medicine to tell them what independent research means to you.

December 20, 2011

Notes

1. To read more about this organization and the report, follow these links: http://www.iom.edu/; http://www.iom.edu/Reports/2011/Breast-Cancer-and-the-Environment-A-Life-Course-Approach.aspx; and http://www.iom.edu/About-IOM.aspx.

2. See this document at http://www.iom.nationalacademies.org/re ports/2011/Breast-Cancer-and-the-Environment-a-life-course-approach .aspx.

Gloves Off

What the Fuck, Komen?

It seems that Komen couldn't take the intense heat and media attention on this one. They announced this morning that they have reversed their position on funding Planned Parenthood. The decision has changed; Komen leadership hasn't. Nancy Brinker refuses to come clean about what was behind the initial denial of funding. Don't be fooled. Komen is still right-wing.

I swore to myself I would not write about the Susan G. Komen for the Cure Foundation (Komen) again anytime soon. After all, what hadn't been said already? But Komen has stepped way over the line with its defunding of Planned Parenthood's breast cancer services. So here we go.

KFC and Komen: A Warning?

In the spring of 2010, Komen partnered with Kentucky Fried Chicken (KFC) to sell pink buckets of chicken. Nutritionists were outraged: selling unhealthy food to poor people to raise money for breast cancer? Breast Cancer Action launched its What the Cluck? campaign in response, encouraging people to contact both Komen and KFC and tell them what they thought of the partnership. Thousands of people did just that. Even Stephen Colbert got into the act with a riff on the campaign and cause marketing in general.

Komen was so roundly criticized for the KFC partnership that you would think they had learned to be careful when they do things that might catch people's attention. If you thought that, you thought wrong.

What's New: Komen's Planned Parenthood Funding Decision

On January 31, 2012, the world learned that Komen had ceased to fund Planned Parenthood's breast cancer services—that is, providing clinical exams and mammograms for poor women who otherwise lack access to health care. (That Planned Parenthood calls these "preventive" services is, of course, a misnomer: these kinds of services don't prevent anything; if they work, they find breast cancer that is already present.)

People are shocked and upset. They should be. What they should not be, however, is surprised.

A Little Komen History

Anyone who has spent any time looking at how Komen works knows that they are the right wing of the breast cancer movement. They are and they stand for the status quo. They push screening when it's not called for, refuse to acknowledge the limitations of mammograms, support drug companies' positions at the FDA over the interest of patients, and ignore the realities of breast cancer in favor of pink-a-fying everything in sight.

Here's a story you may have missed about Komen. Years ago, advocates and activists realized that they had created a federal breast cancer screening program for poor women that guaranteed screening but no access to treatment if breast cancer was found. A number of groups went to Congress to fix this problem. The Komen organization opposed the bill: if you're the Komen Foundation, health care is not a human right. The bill passed despite Komen's opposition.

The right-wing nature of the Komen operation is a direct result of the politics of its well-known founder, Nancy Brinker. Ms. Brinker is a longtime funder of Republican causes and was a Bush "Ranger" during the George Bush II era, raising thousands of dollars for his election efforts. That money netted her an ambassadorship, followed by the position of Chief of White House Protocol.

So no one should be surprised by the Komen move to stop funding Planned Parenthood. But we should look at the history of Komen's relationship to the anti-abortion movement and take a close look at the explanation they give for their decision, because it doesn't pass the red-face test. In fact, they are undercutting their own mission with this decision.

Abortion and Breast Cancer: A Moral Position as a Conflict of Interest

For years, anti-abortion activists have claimed that abortion is a major cause of breast cancer. Though there is no evidence that this is true—see an article in *The Source*, BCA's newsletter—the claim persists.[1] There have even been laws passed in several states requiring that women seeking abortions be counseled that doing so would increase their risk of breast cancer.

For years, these anti-abortion people have criticized Komen loudly for funding Planned Parenthood. Search the Web for *Komen*, *abortion*, and *breast cancer*, and you'll see what I mean. Not because of the breast care that Planned Parenthood provides, but because the anti-abortion people wrongly contend that Planned Parenthood is an abortion mill.

Why would Komen cave now to these wackos? Because they saw an opening that would get the anti-abortion people off their backs, and they took it.

Komen's Rationale for the Planned Parenthood Decision

Komen spokeswoman Leslie Aun told the press that it wasn't abortion politics that drove the decision. Rather, it was a newly adopted Komen rule that prohibits grants to organizations that are under investigation by any legal authority.

Since that statement, no one from Komen has given a press interview. But in classic Komen style, they released an online video of founder Nancy Brinker "setting the record straight," so they could try to tell their version of events without facing questions. (The video no longer exists online at Komen's Web site.) It's interesting to me that Ms. Brinker calls the accusations "scurrilous." That's usually her mode. Attack the accusers and ignore the underlying issues.

So what's the real story on the investigation that has been used as an excuse to cut off Planned Parenthood funding? It's this: Planned Parenthood is being investigated by Cliff Stearns, Republican congressional representative from Florida. Are you surprised to learn that Mr. Stearns has a perfect anti-abortion voting record? What do you think prompted his investigation of Planned Parenthood? Dollars to donuts it's the abortions they provide.

So Komen adopts a new rule that happens to fall right into the anti-abortion snare set by Cliff Stearns. That's not abortion politics? I'm Fred Astaire.

Komen: Undermining Their Own Mission

Komen, as I have written before, is all about screening for breast cancer (see "Don't Make Promises You Can't Keep—Especially in Health").[2] In their efforts to promote screening, Komen has a particular focus on the medically underserved—that is, women who don't have access to routine health care services.

Planned Parenthood affiliates have provided breast screening services to many thousands of women who would otherwise not have this care. That advances Komen's mission. Who will provide these services now? Komen won't.

The Komen decision was made a day after the Centers for Disease Control (CDC) announced that screening rates for breast cancer were down, especially among poor women.

Komen has undercut not only its own mission but the public's perception of who they are. It's about time.

Don't Just Stand There, Do Something

If you're as outraged as you should be, there is something you can do. Write to the Komen Foundation, and tell them what you think of pulling the funding from Planned Parenthood. And get your friends to do the same. Komen won't talk to the press. Let's talk to Komen.

February 3, 2012

Notes

1. See Jane Sprague Zones's article at http://archive.bcaction.org/index.php?page=newsletter-71a.

2. See the original blog post at Healthy Barbs, http://barbarabrenner.net/?p=32.

Yosemite

We're halfway through our February jaunts and thought we would give a little window into our travels.

Our first trip, as you might recall, was to Portland, Oregon, to celebrate our niece Gavrila's recent graduation from Beloit College. The flights to and from Portland went without a hitch, helped considerably by wheelchair assistance, very kind TSA agents, and wonderful friends who transported us to and from the Oakland airport.

Our visit with our Portland family was lovely. Gavi seems thrilled to have moved on to the postcollege phase of her remarkable young life, and many people came to the wonderful party that her parents threw to celebrate her.

The morning after we returned from Portland, Susie packed up the car and off we went for a five-day visit to Yosemite. The drive was beautiful, as it always is. Barbara got to feed herself in a gas station—the wonders of food consumption through a tube.

At the entry station to the park we were handed a guide to accessibility at Yosemite—a pleasant surprise.

Susie had made sure we had an accessible room at Yosemite Lodge. The room worked pretty well, once we worked out the kinks like the lack of a light switch at the entry door, the absence of reachable electrical outlets, and the placement of bathroom light switches behind the bathroom. Being who we are, we made a list of things we discovered that could be improved for people with disabilities and e-mailed them to the Yosemite staff. We received an encouraging response.

Once we got settled in our room, we hooked up with friends

who were joining us for the week. We spent the days having meals together, playing games, talking, and hiking or walking or sitting in a beautiful place and enjoying the glory of Yosemite. Barbara had the bizarre experience of being asked as she sat in the cafeteria gazing at Half Dome whether she was Congresswoman Gabby Giffords.

One of the reasons we love Yosemite so much is that it's always stunning and never the same. The other reason is that we're reminded here that we are, in the words of Lily Tomlin, specks. Whenever you look up in Yosemite, you're towered over by fabulous granite structures and waterfalls.

Because there was no snow in evidence, Susie got to do a long walk with our friends to Mirror Lake and hiked to the Vernal Falls overlook. Susie and Barbara took a day to drive to favorite spots in the park, walk on the accessible trail to the Lower Yosemite Falls view, and cross the Swinging Bridge (which doesn't swing) across the Merced River.

One of the great things about Yosemite is that it teaches you your limits, whether you are temporarily able-bodied or not so much. Our sixty-year-old-plus friends found the Upper Yosemite Falls trail strenuous (because it is), while Barbara could pull off the trail to a view of Lower Yosemite Falls. There, she could visit the source of her "abundance" inspiration that led to her Hebrew name, Shefa, and was reminded again that the water flows to its source, drop by blessed drop.

Because we are required by Barbara's mobility constraints to move slowly along the paths, we got to see God in a lot of things that we might have missed had we been going faster. We saw squirrels whose tails were longer than their bodies. We saw the lichen patterns on the trees. We saw trees fallen at the edge of the creek, providing natural bridges. We saw the trees in the high country that grow at the edge of the granite precipices that overlook Yosemite Valley. We saw the lone tall tree standing straight on the granite ridge. And we saw magnificent tree snags that had been standing for years. The original trees had fallen or broken, providing shelter and food for other vegetation. And then new trees had grown up around them. A fabulous life cycle.

We're now home for a week before traveling to Smith College. Barbara has a visit to the ALS clinic on Monday. If there is more to report after that, we will. Otherwise, look for another entry here after we get back from the East.

Keep those messages coming. We love hearing from you.
Much love,
Barbara & Susie

February 12, 2012

Smith College Medal

You may recall from a journal entry here that Barbara was informed last year that she was being awarded a Smith College Medal. This honor is given annually to five Smith alums whose life and work exemplify "the value of a liberal arts education." Barbara's was awarded for her work in breast cancer. The catch was that the award would not be made in absentia: Barbara would have to show up and participate in the activities expected of medalists.

The awards are given at an annual convocation of the senior class and others of the Smith College community called Rally Day. Rally Day was originally established at Smith to commemorate the birthday of George Washington, and it still occurs on the Thursday of his birthday week.

Since Barbara had already been diagnosed with ALS when she was notified of the award, she immediately contacted the college about her limitations and needs. The staff at Smith was amazing. They responded in the affirmative to every request for accommodation and kept in touch about Barbara's changing physical capacity and needs.

As a result, we got to spend three wonderful days on the Smith campus, participating in events for the medalists. Barbara always kept Kate handy so she could participate in conversations. Susie was by her side throughout, making sure Barbara could deal with whatever came up. Here's our detailed description of the trip.

We arrived on Tuesday evening. We were met at the airport by a Smith driver and accessible van, with a motorized wheelchair in tow. (Barbara got a lot of practice with the chair, which is good since her power wheelchair is being delivered this week.) We were driven to the accessible Ellen Emerson Suite in Barbara's old dorm, Emerson House. We were met there by a lovely woman from the Development Office at Smith who wanted to be sure that we had everything we needed. This kind of reception set the standard for the rest of our time, and that standard was always met.

The first official event we attended was a Wednesday presentation by one of the medalists. There we connected with Rob Dorit, Barbara's faculty host for the award. It was like old home week, since Barbara had worked with Rob for a number of years on breast cancer education at Smith.

That evening there was a dinner for the medalists and their guests, together with members of the Medal Committee and key faculty at the home of the president, Carol Christ. Each of the medalists was introduced to the gathering by a member of the committee. To Barbara's surprise, she was then expected to say something, so she did, focusing her comments on the honor of the award and the quality of the education she received at Smith.

The next day, Rally Day, started with a breakfast for the medalists (and Susie) with the college president, then rehearsal for the awards ceremony. It was here that Barbara finally got to meet her terrific student host, Nahee Kwak, president of the Class of 2014. After rehearsal there was a lunch for medalists and their guests (who, for Barbara, included her sister Nanci and her husband, Bunky, and her brother Rick and his wife, Barbara) and some faculty and college trustees.

The awarding of the medals took place at an assembly of students, faculty, and staff and was a joyous and raucous occasion.

After the official Rally Day convocation ended, there was a reception. Each medalist was situated at a table where she could meet and connect with the Smith community, especially students. Barbara spent quite a bit of time talking with students and the many friends who had come for the event. She was very impressed with the Smith students. Quite a group of women!

That evening, we hosted a pizza dinner for our family and some friends. We got a good pizza recommendation from one of our van drivers, and a good time was had by all until Barbara's fatigue required an end to a glorious day.

On Friday, Barbara was videotaped for the Smith Web site. Then she spent some time with Smith student government leaders who had asked to meet with her. That was followed with time with various friends and then a little rest before the screening of *Pink Ribbons, Inc.* (about cause marketing tied to breast cancer, a production of the National Film Board of Canada). Barbara had prepared about a fifteen-minute introduction to the film (which she will post as a blog soon). Following the screening, a Q-and-A session was held with Barbara, Samantha King (who wrote the book on which the film is based), and Ellen Leopold (author and breast cancer activist who is also in the film). It was a great capstone to an absolutely terrific Smith experience.

We got back to Emerson House around 10:30 and decided we should try to get to sleep for our early pickup for the airport. Imagine our dismay to be awakened at midnight by a fire alarm! So dressed we got, and out into the chilly night we went. The good news is that we got to chat in the cold with Nahee and one of her friends and say good-bye.

Now we get to be home for a while. It's been a wonderful month of travel and adventure.

Much love,
Barbara & Susie

February 26, 2012

Context Is Everything

Framing the Film Pink Ribbons, Inc.

On February 24, 2012, there was a screening of the documentary Pink Ribbons, Inc. *at Smith College. As the recipient of the Smith College Medal for my work as a breast cancer activist, I gave a talk introducing the film. That speech is presented here as I gave it. Imagine a hall with 150 or so souls on a cold, wet Friday night in Northampton, Massachusetts . . .*

Hello, and thank you for being here this evening.

I want to start with a question: will you please raise your hand if you know someone who has or has had breast cancer?

As you will see in the film, if you raised your hand, you are certainly not alone. Almost everyone knows someone with breast cancer. But the other thing you will see in this film is that breast cancer has somehow become good news. Something to celebrate, sing about, dance about, and certainly walk for.

When I had breast cancer at the age of forty-one, I didn't feel like celebrating. What's to celebrate about a life-threatening disease whose treatments amount to—as Susan Love puts it—slash, burn, and poison?

Breast cancer hasn't changed, and its treatments haven't changed that much since I was forty-one, eighteen years ago. And they hadn't changed much for many years prior to my diagnosis either.

There's been some progress on the treatment side, but certainly not enough to jump up and down about. And there's been little if any movement toward true prevention—keeping people from getting breast cancer in the first place—by identifying and eradicating its causes.

What does the general public know about breast cancer? I would argue not much. They know, or think they do, that getting mammograms is the key to beating breast cancer. Some people think mammograms prevent breast cancer, but that can't be true because, when they work, they find cancer that is already there. Mammograms are a detection device, and a far-from-perfect one. Detection and prevention are different. Very different.

The public also knows, or thinks it does, that early detection is the key to survival. But early detection works only for the women whose cancer is both life-threatening when found and treatable with currently available therapies. It isn't necessary for women whose cancer, when found, is not life-threatening, and it doesn't work for women whose cancer, though very small, is so aggressive that it cannot be effectively treated.

And, of course, the public knows that the pink ribbon is the symbol of breast cancer. You'll learn from the film how that came to be, so I won't ruin that story.

People say to me that the pink ribbon—on lapels, on products as varied as toilet paper and handguns—helps raise awareness of breast cancer. My argument is that, thanks in part to the pink ribbon, everyone is now aware of breast cancer, unless they are living under a rock. Isn't it time to move beyond awareness to activism to change the course of the epidemic?

If you think doing a walk for breast cancer, or a run, or a mountain climb is the way to end the breast cancer epidemic, the film you are about to see will, I hope, convince you otherwise.

And if buying a product with a pink ribbon on it would help end the epidemic, it should be over by now, given all the breast cancer shopping that people do. After all, if shopping could cure breast cancer, it would be cured by now.

There is also that "click-on-this-link" kind of activity for funding things like mammograms for poor women. Sounds like a simple and good idea. It is simple, but, like many simple things, it's not so good. It turns out that in 2007, for example, it took five million clicks to fund a total of 129 mammograms. There has to be a better way to provide health care.

As Susan Love says in the film you are about to see, if this is the way we approach breast cancer, we're missing something big. The kind of activism we need is concerned with the larger context, the notion that we should evaluate the messages we get about breast cancer and breast cancer awareness in light of the issue of how we approach research and provide health care. It means challenging the corporations and organizations that stand in the way of better lives for women.

One way to raise those challenges is to Think Before You Pink®. This is a campaign that was started in 2002 by Breast Cancer Action, the kick-ass organization I had the privilege of leading for fifteen years. It focuses on cause marketing: the practice of companies putting a pink ribbon on products to try to increase sales of their products. It provides five questions to guide you as you think about these promotions:

- How much money from your purchase actually goes toward breast cancer? Is the amount clearly stated on the package?

- What is the maximum amount that will be donated?

- How are the funds being raised?

- To what breast cancer organization does the money go, and what types of programs does it support?

- What is the company doing to assure that its products are not actually contributing to the breast cancer epidemic?

Let me give you a cause marketing example that's mentioned in the film. It's about KFC, Kentucky Fried Chicken. A couple of years ago, KFC partnered with the Susan G. Komen for the Cure Foundation. For every pink bucket of fried chicken that KFC sold, they promised to give fifty cents to Komen. Here's the hitch. In case you didn't know, KFC food is really not good for you. And it's sold mostly in economically poor neighborhoods where better food options are hard to find. A lot of nutritionists pointed out this problem and threw up their hands about what could be done about it.

Breast Cancer Action knew what to do about it. We started a campaign to get people to contact KFC and Komen and tell them what they thought of the campaign. We called it "What the Cluck?"

Thousands of people took action. While Komen raised a lot of money from the KFC campaign, they didn't come very close to their $8 million goal, and they took a lot of flak from former supporters about the partnership. KFC was not willing to take that kind of heat two years in a row. They are no longer a Komen partner.

There are other examples in the film. I'll let the movie tell those stories, but keep an ear tuned for the rBGH and General Mills tale in the film. It speaks to the power of ordinary people to create meaningful change.

Not covered in the film is the controversy that was in the news for many days a few weeks ago, involving Komen and Planned Parenthood. In case you missed the brouhaha, it involved a decision by Komen to stop funding Planned Parenthood to do breast care services like breast exams and referrals for mammograms. Komen claimed there weren't politics involved. Instead, they said they had a new policy not to fund any organization that was under investigation. It so happened that Planned Parenthood was the only organization that Komen was funding that fell under this new guideline.

Turns out that Planned Parenthood is under investigation by an anti-abortion Republican congressman who was encouraged to go after the organization by a pro-life group that is furious that Planned Parenthood does abortions.

When the news of the Komen decision became public, a firestorm of public opinion erupted. People complained that women's health was being politicized, that Komen was undercutting poor women who get health care at Planned Parenthood, and that Komen had taken sides in the abortion debate, which has nothing to do with its mission.

Komen responded to the public outcry by claiming its move was not political and then reversing its decision, agreeing to continue funding Planned Parenthood this year.

End of story? Not so fast. The move by Komen and the public outcry in response to it revealed some other things about the breast cancer organization that are now under scrutiny. Like the fact that Nancy Brinker, the founder of Komen, told one story and then another explaining the Planned Parenthood decisions, neither of which made sense. Like the connections of the leadership of Komen to

Republican political candidates and causes. Like the proportion of money that Komen gives to breast cancer research has been declining (to 15 percent of its budget) as their revenues have increased. Like the support given to Komen by selling pink handguns. Like Komen's denial of the toxicity of BPA (Bisphenol A), even though studies have shown that BPA interferes with the effectiveness of some breast cancer treatments. The list is growing.

What surprised me was that people were shocked that women's health was being politicized by the Komen decision. Women's health has always been political, because it's about women struggling to get what they need for their health from a system designed by men for the needs of men.

Breast cancer is no exception. Breast cancer has been political since people noticed years ago that the disease—which primarily affects women—got far less research funding than cancers that primarily affect men. That isn't the case any longer, but it's where the politics of breast cancer started.

Since then, and in many ways because of that effort to increase funding for breast cancer research, a breast cancer movement has come into existence. Like all movements, the breast cancer movement covers a spectrum—from left to right or right to left, depending on where you want to start.

One way to think about the different ends of the spectrum is to consider the kinds of questions that organizations ask at either end.

Toward the right end of the spectrum, groups ask questions like these:

- How can we get more money into breast cancer research?

- Are there drug companies that we can partner with to advance our mission?

- Are there scientists who are willing to tell us what direction breast cancer research should take?

- Are there corporate partners who will fund our work?

- Is there good news on breast cancer for which we can take credit?

Toward the left end of the spectrum, groups ask questions like these:

- With all the money that has been invested in breast cancer research, shouldn't we have better treatments and know more about the causes of breast cancer?

- Will individuals fund our work if we refuse to take money from companies that profit from cancer?

- What direction do people affected by breast cancer want the research to take?

- What are the strengths and weaknesses of the latest research study, and what does it really mean for patients?

- What companies are making products that may increase the risk of breast cancer and how can we organize people to get them to stop?

Some of this spectrum is evident in the film you are about to see. If you think critically, as Smith has taught us to do, about the breast cancer issue, you'll never see a pink ribbon the same way again. Enjoy the film.

February 27, 2012

Choices

How I Live with ALS

At every turn in our lives, we're faced with choices. When I was diagnosed with ALS in November 2010, little did I know about the choices I would be facing. But here I am, making them. Part of my ability to make choices is about resources: money, care providers, and my medical team come to mind. But I think more of my choices are about my attitude.

I think there are essentially two ways of facing any life-threatening or fatal illness: surrendering to it, or trying to manage it. Since surrendering is not my usual m.o., I'm not surprised that I'm trying to manage it to the extent I can. Controlling it is out of the question until research develops treatments that work.

Here are four examples of my approach to ALS. They involve the use of technology to talk, a feeding tube, a neck brace, and wheelchair.

Technology Talks

My ALS is characterized by what is called bulbar onset. That means it first affected the muscles of my mouth and throat. My first symptom was slurred speech. Then it became hard for me to project my voice. With the help of Amy Roman, a fabulous speech therapist at the Forbes Norris Clinic where I'm seen for ALS, I learned about a microphone and amplifier to project my voice. (For information on this technology, see my blog post "There's That Person with . . . ," April 26,

2011.) Maybe I looked funny walking down the street with a mike in front of my mouth, but at least I could be heard.

As my speech continued to deteriorate, and again with advice from Amy Roman, I learned about free text-to-speech programs that speak for me. I type; the software speaks what I type. (For more on this technology, see "Having a Voice, Communicating, and Somewhere in Between," June 17, 2011.)

Is it perfect? Not by a long shot. But, for me, it is way better than being silenced or struggling to make what is left of my ability to speak understood. A choice.

A Feeding Tube Sooner Rather Than Later

The weakness in the bulbar muscles means that I developed trouble swallowing liquids and food. While not everyone with ALS will develop problems swallowing, many will. There are two big problems that accompany problems with swallowing: the risk of choking and the risk of aspirating small bits of food or liquid into your lungs and developing pneumonia. Neither is a pretty picture.

As my swallowing got worse, it took me longer and longer to eat a meal, and choking was a common occurrence. Rather than wait until I ended up in the hospital with pneumonia, I decided I should get a feeding tube.

It's called a PEG (percutaneous endoscopic gastrostomy) tube. It's a tube in my stomach that comes out through a hole just above my belly button. At the end of the tube is a port through which liquid nutrition (and medication, and alcohol or coffee or tea) enters the tube and then my stomach. The nutrition I get is a liquid that comes in a can. (And it's a prescription, so my food is paid for by Medicare.) To maintain my weight, I consume five and a half cans of this stuff a day. And I also take in water through the tube to stay hydrated.

It's not as much fun as eating was by a long shot, but eating had ceased to be fun for me by the time I decided to get the tube. But I can nourish myself (at least for now) and can do it discreetly even in restaurants when we're out with friends. Have tube, will travel.

I could have waited until something dire happened that forced me to get a tube. But, for me, getting the tube before that was a much better approach. It leaves me—for now at least—in control of my food intake and without the risk of something awful happening.

Holding My Head Up

Seems that some of my muscles that are not getting the nerve messages they need to work right are the muscles that allow me to lift my head after I bend over. I had two choices here: go around with my eyes focused on the ground a lot, or get a neck brace to help me hold my head up.

There is a terrific physical therapist at the Forbes Norris Clinic, Michelle Mendoza. I'm at the clinic every three months. The last time I was there, in February, I asked to talk to Michelle. I explained my issue, and Michelle had several approaches for dealing with it. She discussed them with me and showed me the devices and let me try them on.

Since that day, I wear a neck brace most of the time during the day. It helps keep my head from falling too low on my chest, so my muscles don't have to work so hard to lift my head.

Is it fun? No. Does it help? Yes. I imagine that some people don't want to consider solutions like these because they don't like the way it looks. But I would rather look a little out of the ordinary and be able to function as well as I can as long as I can. Choice made.

Wheelchair Assistance

As I type this blog, I'm sitting in a wheelchair at my desk. I don't use the wheelchair all the time, because I don't need to. So why do I have it?

Walking has become more difficult for me over time. I can still walk, usually with the assistance of a walker with wheels, but it's tiring because it requires so much effort to do it. So, when I get tired, I take to my wheelchair. It minimizes fatigue. It's that simple.

I also wanted to learn how to use a motorized chair before I had to be in it all the time—that is, before I'm no longer able to walk. The chair has lots of bells and whistles: the seat elevates and tilts, the back reclines, the footrests extend. I have to learn how to back into our elevator without hitting the walls and how to navigate corners. There's a lot to learn.

I know some people don't want to be in wheelchairs if they don't have to be. I guess the question is what is meant by "have to be." I have to be if I want to conserve my energy and be as high functioning as I can be for as long as I can be. I didn't need to wait until I took a serious fall to think about a wheelchair.

Managing versus Surrendering

Barring a medical miracle or a tornado hitting our house, ALS will get me one day. But, until that day comes, I will work to manage what I can. Using aids like the ones I describe here enables me to continue to function at the level my energy permits. I have a lot to live for and a lot to do. Surrender is not an option for me.

March 16, 2012

Thoughts on Leadership—
Listen Up, Nancy Brinker

My topic this week is not directly related to health. But it concerns a subject very important to all of us who care about health: what to expect from the leaders of our health organizations.

Several things inspire me to write on this topic: my reputation as a leader in the health field, a message I received from someone who taught leadership development, requests I've received lately to get involved with various ALS organizations, and recent developments at the Susan G. Komen for the Cure Foundation.

The Privilege of Leading

Not all of us can lead. Not all of us want to lead. But those of us who have the capacity and the desire must also recognize that leading is a privilege, not a right. We are given this privilege when people are willing to follow us and willing to entrust institutions or organizations they care about to our control.

When people lose faith in leaders, or begin to question their integrity or approach, the privilege of leadership disappears. The privilege of leading means being accountable.

Knowing When to Leave

When I was a teenager there was a popular song that had the lyrics "You got to know when to hold 'em, know when to fold 'em, know when to walk away, know when to run." The song is ostensibly about a card game, but also about life, and it came to mind as I was thinking about leadership. I think there are lessons here.

As applied to the concept of leadership, the song indicates the importance of knowing when it's time to step aside and let others lead. I thought long and hard about when it would be wise for me to step down from the leadership at Breast Cancer Action. I decided that I shouldn't stay at the organization's helm past the age of sixty because BCA's style of activism requires young people, and younger people should lead.

Of course, ALS trumped my retirement plans, but I had announced my intention to retire before that happened.

My thoughts about stepping down from leadership at BCA were driven by my concerns for the organization's future. Leaders think about who they lead—it's to those people that they are responsible.

Maintaining Principles

Leaving a leadership position doesn't mean that leaders stop being leaders. Leaders are teachers: they show people ways of moving forward on issues of concern to them.

Because I was well known in breast cancer, there has been interest in my ALS experience that has led to several articles about me: one in *USA Today* and one recently in the *San Francisco Chronicle*. Each article prompted people from ALS organizations to contact me about getting involved with them.

I have been very cautious about saying yes. That's partly because I have a disease that will increasingly limit my function. But it's also partly because I have principles as a leader in health advocacy that I am not willing to compromise. I evaluate every opportunity through that lens. And, so far, I choose to be independent of any ALS organization; instead, I say what I need to in my blog or in Facebook groups of ALS patients.

Having made these points, I turn to Nancy Brinker's leadership at Komen.

Message to Nancy Brinker at Komen: Time for You to Go

There have been a number of stories in the press over the past week or so about high-level staff members leaving the Komen Foundation in the wake of the Planned Parenthood fiasco. The first to go was Karen Handel, but it was clear then that she was taking the fall for others who had at least as much responsibility. The recent departures reflect to some degree the depth of the problem at Komen.

At the Dallas headquarters, the executive vice president and chief marketing officer, Katherine McGhee, the vice president of global networks, Nancy Macgregor, and the director of affiliate planning and strategy, Joanna Newcomb have all departed or announced their intentions to do so.

In New York, the head of the Komen affiliate announced her resignation. That affiliate also canceled two major fund-raising events because of the concern about the fund-raising climate for the organization in this environment.

Most of these staffers have been with Komen for a long time.

In many places, donations for Race for the Cure participation is down. Way down. The Komen organization is in big trouble.

The message is clear, or should be, to Nancy Brinker, who has been the moving force behind Komen since its inception: people are no longer willing to follow you. Your leadership is at an end.

But Ms. Brinker doesn't seem to be responsible to anyone at the organization. The small board of directors is handpicked by her. The most recent move there is that the current chair is stepping down from the leadership of the board and being replaced by someone close to Brinker. As a friend pointed out to me recently, leaders who are unaccountable to anyone are called dictators. For a handpicked board to express its "complete confidence" in Nancy Brinker says more about the board and its lack of understanding of the harm done to Komen than it does about Brinker's current leadership.[1] When a leader puts personal interests ahead of organizational ones, she not only loses her leadership role but jeopardizes the organization as well. To have an organization as large and as influential as Komen and not be able to think about the organization first is, in my view, a failure of leadership.

For the good of Komen and for all of those who care about ending the breast cancer epidemic, Nancy Brinker should resign and so should the Komen board of directors.

I'm sure Nancy Brinker can find other ways to contribute to the breast cancer cause. If I can with ALS, surely she can with a disease to which she has devoted so much of her time and energy.

If you think Nancy Brinker should resign, tell her so.

March 25, 2012

Note

1. See the article at http://www.reuters.com/article/2012/03/24/us-usa-komen-funding-idUSBRE82M17Y20120324.

Point Reyes

As reported recently, we bought a van that permits us to take Barbara's wheelchair to places we want to go. We thought we would provide an update on the recent van adventures.

The van is a used (2008 with eleven thousand miles) Honda Odyssey, modified for wheelchair use. It has a side door that opens automatically, with a ramp that then folds down to the curb. It also has a kneeling feature to get the ramp to the proper angle for chair access. The other nifty feature is a locking system for the wheelchair, which permits Barbara to ride in her chair in the front passenger position.

As some of you know, we live on a very steep hill. If the van is parked on the hill, it means the ramp is slanted and the wheelchair will have to be tilted to get into it. We tried that a couple of times, but Barbara found it daunting and Susie found it a little heart-stopping. So we park on the flat street above our house and take the theatrics out of getting the wheelchair into the van. The only adventure now is turning the chair from the garage onto the hill.

When we first got the van, we decided we should make sure the locking system for the wheelchair was working. It wasn't. Once we got that fixed, we were ready to travel.

Our first trip was a short one: to the San Francisco premier of *Pink Ribbons, Inc.* That adventure went off without a hitch. So we thought we would go wild and take a day trip to Point Reyes National Seashore this past weekend.

But Barbara discovered that—somewhere, somehow—a screw had been sheared off the control arm for the wheelchair, making it a little dicey to manipulate. So Susie donned her new "wheelchair repairperson" hat, located a new screw, and fixed it. Necessity is, indeed, the mother of invention.

Sunday morning dawned sunny and beautiful. Since there was a break in the rain, we took off for Point Reyes. This is a place that we visited often—typically twice a month—when we first moved to San Francisco in the mid-1970s. We have hiked many of the trails and driven every paved road in the park.

But it's not just the park that is the draw. One of the routes into the park is a beautiful road called Lucas Valley. It passes into western Marin County along streambeds, beautiful hills, a lovely redwood forest, the charming town of Nicasio, and the Nicasio Reservoir. The drive alone is worth the trip. It's the sort of environment that has us marveling periodically, "We live here!"

We got to the park by early afternoon and decided to check in at the visitor center to see about wheelchair-accessible locations. We stopped in the bathroom at the center. It had an accessible stall, but the sinks were too high and the soap dispenser was out of reach from a chair.

To get into the visitor center, a person in a wheelchair needs someone to open the doors, because there is no option to open them electronically. Before we left the park, Susie wrote a comment to the National Park Service about this issue and the bathroom accessibility concerns. Boy, do we see the world through a whole new lens!

We headed out to the paved half-mile earthquake trail, which passes through a lovely meadow, across a stream, through woods, and along the path of the 1906 earthquake—that is, the San Andreas Fault—as it passed through the town of Olema. Birdsong was everywhere. Because Barbara was zipping along in her wheelchair, Susie thinks she's never hiked that trail as fast as we did that day.

We then drove out to the lighthouse along the length of the Point Reyes peninsula, past fabulous waves on the north and south beaches, and passing through the cow ranches that have been active in the area for many generations. While the stairs to the lighthouse prohibited us from getting that far, we did spend time marveling at the Pacific Ocean from the path above the lighthouse.

We stopped for a few minutes at the north beach of the park to watch the waves and then headed back to the visitor center. While we sat there, we saw a magnificent great blue heron coming in for a landing and a bunch of California quail that seemed to be having a marvelous time hanging out.

There are many things to appreciate in God's creation, even when you can't hike.

Much love,
BB & SL

April 2, 2012

Changing the Culture of Health Care in a Consumer Society—Not So Easy

On April 4, 2012, there was a lot of excitement in the press about the fact that nine different boards of medical specialists are now recommending that doctors do fewer tests on patients. The specialties include family practitioners, cardiologists, radiologists, and cancer specialists. Though recommendations to do less testing have been made before and intensely resisted (note the U.S. Preventive Services Task Force recommendation in 2009 to do less mammography screening) for some reason, the fact that medical specialists are making the suggestion now stimulates hope that change will happen. I'm not so sure. Here's why.

The Culture of Health Care in the United States

You may have noticed that in this country we seem to approach health care like other commodities: I need or want it, and I'm going to get it. There's a reason we're referred to as health care "consumers." (Some years ago, Fran Visco of the National Breast Cancer Coalition labeled women with breast cancer as "breast cancer consumers." Don't try to dissect the phrase; you won't like what you find.) People who have resources, who are driving the high cost of medical care, see health care as a thing they are entitled to have, no matter what it costs or whether it has more benefits than risks. And "health care" has come to include all of the tests, drugs, and procedures that might be available to address a medical issue.

This culture has been helped considerably by the Internet, where patients can find information on all sorts of medical care that might or might not work. And the culture has become so ingrained that doctors now fear medical malpractice lawsuits when they decline to order a test or a drug that a patient wants.

Will doctors refuse to prescribe a drug or a test that a patient is demanding just because their specialty group has said, "Don't do it"? I doubt it, because the consequences of not prescribing the thing are much more concrete than what might happen to the doctor if s/he ignores the specialty group's recommendation. If you were a doctor, would you fear more the patient's complaint (and even lawsuit) or the knowledge that you are going against your medical specialty's recommendation, possibly justifying your behavior on the grounds of precaution?

The Role of Patient Advocacy Groups

The cultural drivers toward more and more care are supported by many health advocacy groups focused on specific diseases. From the breast cancer organizations that urge frequent mammograms, to the prostate cancer groups that insist that a PSA (prostate-specific antigen) test will save your life, to the lung cancer groups urging screening with spiral CT scans, to the osteoporosis organizations urging annual bone density tests and pills to address risk rather than disease, the push for more interventions is unrelenting.

Often, these groups receive funding from the drug companies or device manufacturers that sell the things (medication, devices, testing equipment, lab facilities) required for the interventions the groups promote. In other settings, this would be a conflict of interest.

Don't think for a moment that groups whose existence is premised on a belief in a medical test will go quietly away if doctors try to do less of that test. The outcry every time there is a call for less mammography or less PSA testing is a testament to the power of these organizations to mobilize people to protect their turf.

Role of Industry

Another driver of the health care consumer culture in this country is found with the companies that make drugs and medical devices. You are well aware that they are in the business of making money. One of the ways they do that is by getting consumers to demand things of their doctors. They do this by advertising their products to consumers. Direct-to-consumer advertising of drugs, which has been happening in the way it is now in the United States since the 1970s, has helped drive demand for and consumption of medical care off the charts.

One of the reasons patients demand so much of their doctors is that the drug companies tell them to. You know: the ads that end with, "Ask your doctor."

Want to Change the Culture? Ask Different Questions

If you want to change the culture of health care, think about asking different questions like:

- Do I need this treatment? Will it help me? What percentage of patients who receive this treatment benefit from it? How great is the benefit? What are the risks?

- Is the test or treatment my doctor is recommending one I need? What's the purpose of this test or treatment? Does it address a condition I have?

- Is the advocacy group that's recommending this device funded in part by the manufacturer?

- Is my congressional representative committed to ending direct-to-consumer drug advertising?

The doctors alone can't change the culture. We all have to do it.

April 14, 2012

Whatever Happened to Previews of Coming Attractions in Health?

Anybody who knows about ALS knows where those of us with the disease end up. But there are steps along the way that can be anticipated and, if anticipated, dealt with to minimize discomfort. As I thought about my own situation recently, I realized that there are lots of ways the medical profession could help people if they would just communicate about what's coming.

And I don't mean doctors saying what they think will happen up ahead, as doctors sometimes do. We all know, don't we, that doctors are just people with particular training that doesn't include training in clairvoyance?

But there are things medical people actually know that it would be helpful if they communicated. Here are a few examples of how that might work. All are taken from my own experience or the experience of friends.

What Happens to Your Feet When You Can't Walk So Much?

A couple of weeks ago, my feet started swelling up. When the swelling didn't go away, I e-mailed the terrific nurse at the Forbes Norris Clinic, where I'm seen for ALS, and asked what might explain it. The answer was dependent edema, when fluid builds up in appendages that are mostly idle. It's like being on a twenty-five-hour airplane ride. So as ALS progresses in the legs, making it harder to walk, ALS patients like me walk less, and their feet swell.

While I was distressed by the symptom, I was more unhappy that no one had told me that it might occur or what could be done either to prevent it or make it go away. Turns out that a pretty straightforward lymphatic massage that my yoga instructor/Thai masseuse suggested is really quite helpful for reducing the swelling. And the clinic nurse knew about feet and ankle exercises to reduce the risk of swelling.

If we know that dependent edema happens, and we know it happens in people who stop walking much, and we know that people with ALS stop walking much, why don't we tell them that it might happen and give them the tools to minimize it and treat it if it does occur? The medical profession should not make the patients come to them complaining about things that can be anticipated. We have enough on our hands.

When Is It Useful for People with ALS to Record Their Voices?

People with ALS lose the ability to talk because the muscles that control speech stop working. Sometimes this is how ALS first manifests. It's called bulbar onset.

Fortunately, some speech pathologists devote their lives to helping ALS patients. They know a lot of things. One thing they seem to know is that there are ways to record your voice while you still have it so that the sounds can be used in text-to-speech programs that exist.

Of course, this is only possible while a patient can still talk reasonably well. By the time I was told about this option, I wasn't one of them. Information that might have been very helpful if given in a timely manner.

How Long Does It Take to Recover from Abdominal Surgery?

Abdominal surgery isn't rare; a lot of it is done every year. As a result, there's a lot of experience that can tell us how long, on average, patients take to recover from the surgery to the point where they feel like their normal selves. So why don't surgeons tell patients how long it will be?

A friend of mine recently had emergency abdominal surgery for an intestinal adhesion. Very scary. After the surgery, her surgeon told her that she could go back to work in a few weeks and said not one word about how long her recovery time would be. The medical excuse for her to explain her absence from work was only good for those few weeks.

If a doctor tells you that you can go back to work two weeks after surgery, isn't it rational to expect that time frame to bear some relationship to recovery time from the surgery? In fact, it was nearly six weeks before my friend began to feel recovered. Is it that the doctor didn't know or that he just wasn't telling? Either answer is simply unacceptable.

Does a Double Mastectomy Reduce Your Risk of Breast Cancer to Zero?

We know the answer to this one, and it's "no." Because we have much more breast tissue than mastectomies can remove, there remains a small but measurable risk of breast cancer even after the surgery.

I heard recently about a woman who asked her oncologist this question, clearly hoping that the answer was "yes." Indeed, that's the answer the doctor gave. I know this oncologist, and I know he knows that his answer was wrong. Whom did he think he was protecting? Why is the truth so hard to tell?

Duty to Warn?

Each of these examples points to a failure in the medical community both to realistically anticipate and communicate with patients about conditions or situations that can be easily anticipated. In the legal system, there's a duty to warn people who might reasonably come in contact with dangerous products or conditions that those dangers exist. Doesn't the medical community have the same duty? Shouldn't it?

May 10, 2012

Susan Love

Time to Think before You Pink

There are many heroes and heroines in the world of breast cancer. You even know some of their names. One of the best known is Dr. Susan Love, author of *Dr. Susan Love's Breast Book*, the excellent layperson's guide to breast cancer issues. I have given that book to several people and referred many others to it as a clear and invaluable source of information for sorting out questions about breast cancer diagnoses and options for treatment.

Dr. Love stopped doing surgery some years ago and now runs a foundation, called—you can guess it from the title of her book—the Susan Love Breast Cancer Foundation. Founded in 1995, its mission is "to eradicate breast cancer and improve the quality of women's health through innovative research, education, and advocacy." According to its latest annual report, the foundation has nearly five million dollars in assets.

Eradicating breast cancer was not always the foundation's stated mission. In 2005, its stated mission was "to end breast cancer in ten years." I was then the executive director at Breast Cancer Action and had heard similar elusive promises from others many times. But I thought of Susan as more honest than most people in the field, so I was surprised. I e-mailed her to ask from what year we should start counting the ten years. She responded, "My board says when we raise all the money." Oh, yeah, the money thing. As 2015 approaches, the mission has changed. Either they didn't raise all the money they needed or they saw that they couldn't deliver. Surprise.

I have known Susan Love a long time and—despite her excellent book—disagreed with her about several things along the way. When we first "met" in 1994 at an online breast cancer forum, we disagreed about the value of breast self-exam. We still disagree about that. Susan says it sends women on a fearful "search and destroy" mission that doesn't do any good. I say that discouraging women from knowing their own bodies is a dangerous thing, especially when about one-third of women with breast cancer find their own lumps.

But more recent events have intensified my disagreements with her. Here's why.

Both Susan and I appear in the film that's opening now across the country, *Pink Ribbons, Inc.* In that film, Susan convincingly says we have to find the cause of breast cancer and stop it. In the film, she eloquently suggests that environmental research may be the key and that people who want to support that kind of research should be sure that's where their money is going. It's clear to me that this call is for more funding for her foundation.

So far, so good, right? But Susan can't really be that interested in environmental causes of breast cancer, because if she were she couldn't accept some of the funding the foundation has accepted or establish partnerships the foundation has established.

I suspected as much when the foundation announced to great fanfare its "Army of Women" approach to getting women involved in breast cancer studies. The Army was launched with the help of funding and publicity from the Avon Foundation.

I was also pretty sure that the partnership was a direct result of the fact that Love was serving on the Avon Foundation's Breast Cancer Scientific Advisory Board at the time. If you don't think this is how funding works, think again. Look at the list of who serves on a nonprofit research funder's advisory board, and see if you don't find many of those names also on the list of the funder's grantees.

So what's the problem? Avon (the corporate parent of the Avon Foundation) refuses to sign on to the Campaign for Safe Cosmetics (http://safecosmetics.org/) and continues to use known or suspected carcinogens in some of their products. This corporate hypocrisy is also highlighted in *Pink Ribbons, Inc.*

My suspicions about Susan's commitment to environmental

health research were confirmed recently when Susan announced with great pride that her foundation has been chosen to benefit from the Ford Motor Company's Ford Warriors in Pink Models of Courage campaign. The foundation will get the "net proceeds" (that means after costs are covered, so it could be little or nothing) of sales of things like Warriors in Pink T-shirts, yoga pants, and sun hats, to name a few items. You can array yourself in much Ford Warrior in Pink apparel.

The Ford Motor Company is also featured in *Pink Ribbons, Inc.* Ford has a history of being the leading polluter in the automotive industry. And we know that some of the things that are produced by internal combustion engine cars can increase the risk of many cancers, including breast cancer. Beyond that, the film includes a sequence that focuses on the elevated incidence of cancer in women who worked in automotive plastics factories, making parts for Ford. Ford's purported concern about breast cancer is classic pinkwashing. And Susan Love is helping them do it. For shame.

Susan says in the film that she hates pink. But she partners with companies that are pinkwashers. Will the real Susan please stand up?

I invite you to join with me in calling on Susan Love to run her foundation with the same integrity she exhibited in *Dr. Susan Love's Breast Book.*

June 5, 2012

❧

Who Shall Live and Who Shall Die?

A Yom Kippur Reflection

This past week marked the end of what we Jews call the Days of Awe, the ten days between Rosh Hashanah, the Jewish New Year, and Yom Kippur, the Day of Atonement, which is the holiest day in the Jewish calendar. Susie, my beloved partner, and I attended services at the Mendocino Coast Jewish Community, where we have been members for many years. This year, our friend and rabbi Margaret Holub asked me to do a teaching on a prayer that we say at Yom Kippur called the Unataneh Tokef. The prayer's most famous lines, at least to Jews, are: "On Rosh Hashanah it is written, on Yom Kippur it is sealed, . . . who shall live and who shall die. . . ."

The Days of Awe are so named because during the time between Rosh Hashanah and Yom Kippur Jews are called on to examine their lives, their relationships with people, and their relationship with God. They are called to turn, through these examinations, toward God.

Below is the text of the talk I gave on Yom Kippur.

Thoughts on Unataneh Tokef

Our High Holiday *mohzor* (prayer book) is filled with reminders—as if we needed to be reminded—that life is cyclical. As Emmylou Harris sings, "We are all born to live; we are all bound to die."

Some of these reminders are relatively gentle. That cannot, however, be said of the best known part of Unataneh Tokef, a prayer that many of us know at least a part of by heart. That part is: "On Rosh

Hashanah it is written, on Yom Kippur it is sealed, how many will leave this world and how many shall be born into it, who shall live and who shall die. . . ."

After a long litany of the many ways we might die, we are told that, while we cannot change the decree, *tshuvah* (turning), *tefillah* (study), and *tzedakah* (charity) will make our fate easier.

If tshuvah, tefillah, and tzedakah could reverse the decree, I suspect the world would already be filled with many more devout and very old Jews.

I think it's odd that this prayer is a central part of the Yom Kippur liturgy, because by the time it rolls around, it's time for the ledger to be sealed and may be too late to do anything about it. At the same time, I don't find any indication in the mohzor that what is written on Rosh Hashanah ever changes by the time Yom Kippur arrives. Nonetheless, like others more steeped in our tradition than I am, I have been struggling to understand what this prayer means, how to take it in.

I wonder if anyone still believes that God actually has a ledger book in which all our names appear and that God makes an entry each year for each of us. But even if we don't believe this, this prayer captures our attention and imagination, prompting us to wonder and pray that we end up on the living side of the ledger on Yom Kippur.

Because of this hope, it is during these days of awe that we ask ourselves questions about how we live our lives, ask whether our lives have purpose and meaning. Yom Kippur drives us to examine our lives, not because we're necessarily going to die in the next year, but because doing so may result in tshuvah—turning toward God. Since we can't know (not even I know despite my illness) whether we are written and sealed for another year, we strive to turn toward God so that, whenever our time comes, we have done our best to lead meaningful lives.

In a perfect reflection of Judaism, I think that what's important in the Days of Awe are the questions we ask ourselves, not necessarily the answers to those questions. Because questions prod us to examine ourselves and our lives deeply. The questions aren't just for the Days of Awe; they are for every day.

It's not about getting to heaven, especially if you don't believe there is one. It's about examining ourselves to be sure we are living our lives to the fullest, with purpose and meaning. I think this is part of what [Rabbi] Margaret was talking about in her *drash* (interpretation of text) on Erev Rosh Hashanah (the evening service of Rosh Hashanah). While being inscribed in the book of life is a thing to pray for, it's how we live the lives we are given—however short or long—that indicates how we incorporate tshuvah, tefillah, and tzedakah.

The singer-songwriter Kevin Welch, who I doubt is Jewish, has lyrics that go like this: "There'll be two dates on your tombstone. And all your friends will read 'em. But all that's gonna matter is that little dash between 'em."

The poet Mary Oliver, in a poem called "The Summer Day," expresses it a little differently: "Tell me, what is it you plan to do / With your one wild and precious life?"

The point of personal, self-reflective questions is to focus us on how we live now and how we need to change. If we do this, it does not matter a lot whether we're not inscribed this year or next or ten years from now. Because we all die. The question is, are the lives we're leading ones of connection, contemplation, and good deeds?

The poet Rilke offers this, from *Letters to a Young Poet*:

Have patience with everything that is unresolved in your heart.
And try to love the questions themselves. Don't search for the
answers, which could not be given to you now, because you
would not be able to live them. And the point is, to live everything. *Live* the questions now. Perhaps then, someday far in the
future, you will gradually, without even noticing it, live your
way into the answer.

Rilke also offers this poem, which I think speaks to how we live our lives in relationship to God:

God speaks to each of us as he makes us,
then walks with us silently out of the night.

These are words we dimly hear:

You, sent out beyond your recall,
go to the limits of your longing.
Embody me.

Flare up like flame
and make big shadows I can move in.

Let everything happen to you: beauty and terror.
Just keep going. No feeling is final.
Don't let yourself lose me.

Nearby is the country they call life.
You will know it by its seriousness.

Give me your hand.

In this day and age, I think Unataneh Tokef's true significance is not whether God in fact sits in judgment of each of us, but whether we believe that, in some meaningful way, our lives depend on our power to change, to take God's hand, to engage in tshuvah, tefillah, and tzedakah. These things make it easier to bear what God may decree. I think they do so by helping us to live lives of learning, connection, and good deeds that benefit the communities in which we live. That brings us closer to God in all of God's many manifestations.

Since we cannot know where our names appear in the book, maybe the purpose of acknowledging that on Rosh Hashanah it is written and on Yom Kippur it is sealed is to remind us that, whenever and however we die, our obligation is to notice—ourselves, our relationships with others, the good we do in the world. We are finite, but we transcend death by the way we live our lives and connect with each other and with God. The good we do lives on through the lives we've touched.

Life, death, and birth are mysteries that are in God's hands. We cannot control them. But we can control our attitude toward them. I don't think my having ALS is a way that God is punishing me. We're all going to die of something. My challenge is to live whatever life I have left in tshuvah, tefillah, and tzedakah. I think that is the challenge for all of us, even those of us who are perfectly healthy today.

As I explained to someone else with ALS who was asking why I call myself a "practicing Jew," I see myself as constantly striving toward a meaningful life and, through that life, a relationship with God. It's a practice. Some people may get it perfectly right, but I think most of us—myself included—keep working to achieve tshuvah. I think that is the message of Unataneh Tokef.

September 29, 2012

NBCC

The Promise, the Process, and the Problems

I have a reputation as an expert on breast cancer and breast cancer advocacy organizations, gained during my fifteen years as the (now former) executive director of Breast Cancer Action. Since it's once again October—Breast Cancer Industry Month—I thought I should use that expertise to talk about an organization that does a lot of good but seems to be misguided in a couple of important ways. That organization calls itself the National Breast Cancer Coalition, or NBCC.

NBCC promotes nuanced messages about breast cancer, does not overhype treatment news, and encourages an evidence-based approach to treatments. It also encourages people to move beyond breast cancer "awareness," which Lord knows we have enough of.

But despite its name, NBCC does not represent all breast cancer organizations. No group does. It is the brainchild and is under the close control of Fran Visco, its founding executive director and now president. Like many charismatic leaders, Fran surrounds herself with people and groups who agree with her, declining to confer or collaborate with those who disagree or don't sing her praises. Unfortunately, that limits NBCC's effectiveness.

A Breast Cancer Deadline?

NBCC's current focus is on a "deadline" to end breast cancer by January 1, 2020. When they field-tested this campaign with some of the breast cancer researchers with whom they work, they were told in no uncertain terms that setting a deadline would be counterproductive to research. But set a deadline they did.

Of course, they are not the first to set a deadline for solving the breast cancer problem. Susan Love set one in 2005. For what happened to that, see my post "Susan Love: Time to Think before You Pink" (June 5, 2012). And how many times have we been told by doctors and researchers that in the next five or ten years the problem will be solved?

One problem with deadlines is that they assume that you have control over the problem you've identified. NBCC does not have that control. It's an advocacy organization. It doesn't do or fund research, though a lot of researchers work with them. NBCC also doesn't control the legislative agenda for research, try as they might to do so. Under these circumstances, how might they expect to meet their deadline? They have a stated strategy, but it doesn't seem to include working with other groups that know a thing or two about the topics being addressed. The NBCC strategy is: leave it to us.

I also should say that I think ending breast cancer is a promise that no one can keep. Breast cancer has been with us since before the Greeks. I think it will be with us always. The questions are (1) can the incidence be reduced, and (2) can the treatments be improved?

What will happen when January 1, 2020, rolls around and breast cancer persists? I assure that you NBCC will find some other mission to pursue that will allow them to continue to raise funds. Will they acknowledge failure? I doubt it. Barring a miracle, I won't be around to witness that date, but I hope some people who read this will be here and will remember.

NBCC's Legislative Strategy

NBCC has been active in lobbying Congress and has had some success getting bills addressing breast cancer research passed. As far as I know, their efforts have focused on the Department of Defense (DoD) Breast Cancer Research Program, environmental breast cancer research, and, most recently, an Act to Accelerate the End of Breast Cancer.

The DoD program—which drives funding through the DoD:

it does not restrict its funding to the military—is NBCC's longest-standing success.

What all these legislative efforts have in common is a commission of some sort to guide the program efforts. The commissions, set up by the laws for which NBCC advocates, are composed of lay people and scientific experts. The participants are selected with NBCC approval.

These are efforts funded with taxpayer dollars. Why should NBCC and Fran Visco get to decide who the deciders are? Who elected them? And will NBCC veto someone important to the discussions?

Time for New Leadership?

The competition among breast cancer organizations—for funding and for influence—is fierce. It leads to deadlines and promises that can't be met and to steps that are more effective at achieving influence and dominance than at addressing the incidence and treatment of the disease. Witness the Komen Foundation, for example. It's time for leaders who can bring people and organizations together. We need new approaches. In fact, I think the movement needs new leaders.

October 21, 2012

Winter Weather

Winter weather has arrived in San Francisco. We've already had quite a bit of rain, which means we are pursuing more activities that take place indoors. We've never been folks who liked being outdoors in the rain, and that has not changed. Barbara has always loved the rainy season and is pleased to see that the rain does not deter the hummingbirds from feeding at our feeder. Susie would prefer sun.

We had planned to make our annual trip to see the sandhill cranes at Lodi, California, last weekend, but rain made us defer that trip. Instead, we went to the movie *Lincoln*. We give the movie four thumbs up. Daniel Day Lewis left us both feeling we had just seen Abe Lincoln onscreen.

The rain did clear enough for us to make a one-day excursion to Yosemite, a place we love, to meet up with Susie's sister and her husband. On the way, Barbara played DJ while Susie drove through hills that had turned a lovely green with the rain. The winter light was fabulous. There were more clouds and fog than we expected along the way, but all of that cleared about seven miles outside the park, along the beautiful Merced River. We connected with our family, drove to lunch at the Ahwanhee Bar, and then rolled and strolled the accessible path to Lower Yosemite Falls. By that time, there were some clouds evident in the valley that made the views quite beautiful as the setting sun hit them. We were really glad we made the trip.

We talked in a recent post about how helpful it is to have a helper here for Barbara from the Seniors at Home program of Jewish

Family and Children's Services. Nini is here six days a week for two hours and is an enormous help on many fronts.

As Barbara finds it harder to walk, we are taking (figurative) steps to make sure we have all the help we need to face what's happening now and in the future. We have signed up for hospice services through Hospice by the Bay, and we now have a nurse and social worker assigned to us. For the time being, we will meet with our hospice nurse once a week and know that the hospice is on call 24/7 to help us deal with things as they arise. We are also exploring the possibility of having hospice volunteers be with us several times a week to make sure Barbara's needs are met when Susie is out.

You may think of hospice as about end-of-life care, and it is, but that's not all it is. Hospice provides comfort care for people with incurable conditions. We decided to establish a relationship with hospice now, before we're in crisis mode and while we can take advantage of many of the services the program offers.

Barbara is exploring getting more Botox, this time to control excess saliva that is one of the effects of ALS. We'll keep you posted on that.

We had a lovely Thanksgiving with a few friends and hope you enjoyed time with your family and friends. We give thanks for all of you!

Keep those messages coming.

Love,

Barbara & Susie

December 10, 2012

What I Learned as a Volunteer

On Sunday, December 9, 2012, I was awarded the Lola Hanzel Coura-geous Advocacy Award by the American Civil Liberties Union of North-ern California (ACLU–NC) at their annual Bill of Rights Day Celebration. Below is my acceptance speech for the award. I delivered the speech using text-to-speech software on my iPad. I have put in brackets explanatory in-formation for folks who are not familiar with ACLU–NC.

When Mickey Welsh [chair of the ACLU–NC board of direc-tors] e-mailed to tell me that I was to receive this award today, I was incredulous and humbled. I know a lot of the people who have gotten this award in previous years, and I am honored to be included in this august company.

I embarked on my relationship with the ACLU when I volun-teered for the New Jersey affiliate in 1975. Little did I know that the work I did then on prison reform was just the beginning of many years of working with the ACLU.

I won't bore you with all of the volunteer jobs I've had at various ACLU affiliates and the national office—though I think it's important to point out that the ACLU always had the wisdom not to appoint me to a finance committee. What I want to talk about is not how I helped the ACLU, but how I was helped by the many roles I had with the ACLU over time, one of the two organizations that are closest to my heart.

My experience with the ACLU confirms that volunteering is its own reward. I'm sure that my work with the ACLU—as a board member, a legal intern, a member of the legal committee, a member of the board nominating committee, a representative to the Biennial

Conference, a member of the national board, a fund-raiser—was of value to the organization. At the same time, I learned so much—about civil liberties, about justice, about organizing, about effective campaigns, and about how great nonprofits are run—and I met some lifelong friends. At the ACLU, I learned how to be an effective activist. And, much to my surprise, I developed skills that would allow me to be an effective staff leader of another organization.

I was in my third term on the ACLU–NC board (not three consecutive terms, that would be a no-no) [ACLU–NC policy requires board members to cycle off the board after two consecutive terms] when I was diagnosed with breast cancer. I was forty-one years old. While I was in treatment, I resigned from the board and decided to stop practicing law to look for a job in health advocacy.

I ended up as the executive director of Breast Cancer Action, a tiny organization trying to tell the truth about breast cancer. There were already a lot of organizational players making their voices heard with a pretty pink and deeply misleading story. I was the first full-time employee of Breast Cancer Action—or as I referred to it, BCA—with no experience in running or building an organization except what I'd learned at the ACLU. It turned out that that was plenty.

I had learned at the ACLU that an important part of getting your organizational message out was an effective press strategy. And one of my good friends from the ACLU was Elaine Elinson, the mistress of [ACLU–NC] press relations—I think she had a slightly less grand official title. I asked Elaine, who had a connection to breast cancer, to join the Breast Cancer Action board of directors and guide me in a media strategy. That may have been the smartest thing I ever did at BCA.

It was also at the ACLU that I learned about board term limits as a way of balancing board members knowledgeable about organizational history with new people with fresh energy and ideas. We modeled Breast Cancer Action's board term limits on those of ACLU–NC.

I also thought, based on my experience with the ACLU, that having written policy statements was important as a guide for people working for the organization either as staff or volunteers, and as educational tools for others. So I worked with the board to write policies on topics on which Breast Cancer Action was involved.

But the biggest thing I brought to BCA was a social justice

perspective that had been honed through my work with the ACLU. It's a rare issue that can be successfully addressed without understanding the context in which it occurs. But there were no breast cancer organizations operating at the national level that addressed breast cancer through a social justice lens. It was fine to talk about new treatments, but we also needed to focus attention on who could get them and how much that depended on patients being able to find out about them, on the doctors they saw or the clinics they went to, and having money to pay for them.

And the information people got about treatments was often prepared by the drug manufacturer, focusing on the benefits and downplaying the risks.

The talk about differences in breast cancer incidence and mortality among different racial groups is always labeled as a focus on disparities. But disparity just means difference. BCA called these differences inequities and raised questions about the social, cultural, physical, and economic realities of different racial groups that go a long way to explaining the incidence and mortality differences. Only by addressing inequities can we hope to minimize the differences.

When places like Marin County got attention about its high breast cancer rates, Breast Cancer Action would point out that there were a lot of black women dying at young ages in Bayview–Hunters Point that needed at least as much attention.

On the subject of environmental links to breast cancer, BCA called for studying the usually poor communities that are often situated near pollution sources and therefore at highest risk.

When it came to programs providing mammography screening for poor women, Breast Cancer Action took the position that if the government was going to pay for breast screening for poor women, then women diagnosed with the disease should also have their treatment paid for by the government. Remarkably, that was not the law. It is now.

And there were areas where, as the leader of Breast Cancer Action I took a different course from the one that the ACLU national organization had adopted when I was on the board. I had been in the dissenting minority at the national board when I and others urged the organization to endorse limiting corporate contributions in elections. This affiliate [ACLU–NC] endorses these limits. The area of corporate influence in cancer advocacy isn't about elections so much as it is about the reality or the perception that corporations that make drugs and devices for cancer use donations to influence the advocacy that cancer organizations do around treatment issues.

Breast Cancer Action was the first cancer advocacy organization to make it a matter of policy not to accept funding from corporations profiting from cancer or contributing to cancer by environmental harm.

It was the corporate contributions policy that in many ways enabled BCA to have, in a small way, an impact on breast cancer advocacy similar to that of the ACLU on a wide range of civil liberties issues. We launched our Think Before You Pink® campaign in 2002, raising questions about all the products sold with pink ribbons on them. We called for more transparency in these sales efforts. After all, if shopping could cure breast cancer, shouldn't it be cured by now? We also called out "pinkwashers," companies that sold some product to raise money for breast cancer while at the same time making products that were likely contributing to the breast cancer epidemic. There's now a documentary film about the pinking of breast cancer and pinkwashers. It's called *Pink Ribbons, Inc.*, and you saw a clip from it here this afternoon. The film is available on DVD and Netflix.

There's one more area of social justice where Breast Cancer Action's goals overlapped completely with those of the ACLU. That issue is the patenting of human genes, in this case the breast cancer genes known as BRCA-1 and -2. BCA had tried unsuccessfully to get someone in Congress to address this issue when the patents on these two human genes were first issued. When the ACLU started examining the issue, they contacted us, and when the lawsuit was prepared to challenge the patents, Breast Cancer Action was the only national organization to sign on as a plaintiff. We could do that because we didn't accept funding from the patent holder, Myriad Genetics.

Sooner or later, all issues of social justice are connected. And we as individuals can advance the arc of history toward justice by volunteering. The world changes because we work for change. I am deeply grateful for the privilege of volunteering for the ACLU and very honored to be the recipient of this Lola Hanzel Courageous Advocacy Award.

December 13, 2012

January 19, 2013

We've had a couple of lovely California days during the past few weeks. We've also had delightful visits from friends and family from near and far.

There are several changes in our lives related to Barbara's illness. As her ability to balance on her feet lessens and her legs weaken, she has become more prone to falling. So she now spends most of her time in her wheelchair. It's safer, and it gives her more freedom of motion than she was getting recently with her walker. It also means she needs help to get to the bathroom: that transfer from the wheelchair can be treacherous!

In light of Barbara's declining physical condition, we are engaging more people to be here when Barbara would otherwise be home alone. We are so far using our home care person, hospice volunteers, and friends to cover these times. As Barbara needs more help, we will make sure she has all the home health care services she needs.

Fortunately, Barbara can still type better than many of us ever could. And her mind is humming along, as you know if you are her Facebook friend or reader of her blog.

We still get out for rolls and strolls when the weather permits. We get to classical music concerts and plays. We watch lots of movies on DVD—feel free to post movie recommendations or "must miss" films. And we spend time with friends and with each other.

Susie is in charge of all that happens around Barbara's home care. (She always consults Barbara, of course.) She also volunteers at the Magic Theatre, gets to the gym every weekday, and tries to join the Sunday morning hikers on days when we don't have tickets to a matinee.

Thanks so much for messages, your prayers, and your love.
Barbara & Susie

February 11, 2013

It's been about three weeks since we posted a journal entry, so we figure it's time for an update.

Barbara's illness continues to progress; we continue to deal with what comes up and try to anticipate future needs. As we mentioned in an earlier entry, Susie is uncomfortable leaving Barbara alone without someone to help her nourish or go to the bathroom, so we have engaged more time—eight hours a day—from the folks at Seniors at Home. Volunteers from Hospice by the Bay and friends help out when we don't have paid staff and Susie needs to be elsewhere.

A Hoyer Lift—to move Barbara from her wheelchair to bed or to the toilet—now lives in our bedroom (boy, is that room getting crowded!), and Susie knows how to use it. When it becomes impossible for Barbara to transfer herself to bed or to the toilet, Susie will train the home care staff on how to use it.

Barbara got more Botox injections to try to control her mouth secretions. We'll know how effective they were by the end of this week.

We spent last Friday afternoon at the UCSF ALS Clinic. We were both impressed at how engaged all the staff we met with were. They are clearly focused on both extending life and maintaining quality of life. Based on that visit, Barbara will be trying another nutritional formula that the dietician hopes will be more digestible and another drug to try to improve her digestive *motility* (a medical word meaning "ability to move spontaneously"). Though ALS is not thought to affect the digestive tract, the UCSF dietician says they see a lot of patients with this problem. If Barbara's problems with digestion continue despite these changes, there may be a new procedure and tube (a J-tube) in her future.

The physical therapist and occupational therapist were both unexpectedly away on the day we visited the clinic. But Barbara had identified her issues with neck support in a message she sent to the clinic before her visit. The UCSF staff will follow up, and a home visit may be in the works.

On the more fun side of our lives, we've enjoyed rolls and strolls to the Arboretum and the San Francisco waterfront and around the 'hood. We've seen two plays: *Our Practical Heaven* at the Aurora Theatre in Berkeley (pretty good) and *Se Llama Christina* at the Magic Theatre (also pretty good—and, yes, both companies actually spell *theatre* this way. Barbara thinks the spelling is pretentious). We also saw the National Theater live screening of *The Magistrate,* starring John Lithgow. This is a simulcast production of the fabulous British theater. If you are interested, it may be in a theater near you.

We're watching lots of movies. For baseball fans we recommend *Trouble with the Curve,* featuring Clint Eastwood and Amy Adams. For a more reflective movie, we recommend *Of Gods and Men,* a true story about a small group of Catholic monks trying to carry on in civil war-torn Iraq. We are also catching up on television series we missed. We are thoroughly enjoying *Pushing Daisies,* and we're finally catching up to a lot of our friends who are *Downton Abbey* addicts.

We have been blessed with visits from family and friends from near and far. We are delighted to see new blooms on the flowering plum tree we planted out front last year. (The image that accompanies this blog isn't our tree, but we hope—and expect—ours will look like this in a few days.) And Barbara has spotted a few hummingbirds just sitting for a very long time on the hummingbird feeder. She wonders if that's a sign of an aging hummingbird. Anyone know?

We treasure your friendship, your love, and your messages.

Love,

Barbara & Susie

Thanks and Blessings

As my life comes to an end, I want to thank readers of this blog and our Caring Bridge site for reading all that I have written while I deal with ALS. I'm sure some of what I wrote was difficult to read, some of what I wrote helped others, while other pieces just made you think. This blog will be up a while—and some ambitious person might turn it into a book. If you think of others who might benefit from anything I've written, please send it along to them.

I have been blessed to lead a rich life, full of love and culture and travel and work that had meaning for me. I have no regrets except that I got ALS in the first place.

I have met amazing people both in person and online. Everyone I have come in contact with has had something unique to offer the world. The world is a better place because these people are or were in it. Some of these people I have mentored (and you know who you are); others have taught me. What I know about all of these people is that I have been blessed to know them and that they will succeed at what they set their hearts and minds to do.

In the Jewish tradition there is a Priestly Blessing. I copy it here because it is what I wish for all readers of these words:

> May the Lord bless you
> and keep you;
> May the Lord make his face shine on you
> and be gracious to you;
> May the Lord turn his face toward you
> and give you peace.

May 7, 2013

Anne Lamott

God, I loved Barbara Brenner, and still do. She taught me through the years how to be both a more radical and a more tender activist and woman. And wow, what a way with words, a writer after my own heart.

I was frequently the emcee of Breast Cancer Action symposiums and galas, and she and Susie Lampert came to be my beloved friends. Side by side at all those events, we offered images of our beloved friends and family members who had died of breast cancer, and we cried for their passing and cheered for their lives. We offered them up so that they would never be forgotten and so that they would always live here with us in many ways—gone only in one. Arms linked, in circles, we refused as a radical act to let anyone convince us that we should get over anyone's loss, ever, if we didn't feel like it.

And Barbara never, ever gave up on anyone. She scrambled and nudged and roared at people who could give knowledge, support, medicine, and hope to the living.

Over the years I watched Barbara grow from a passionate advocate and organizer into a hugely spiritual woman and teacher and guide. She made other people look at the faces of those we had lost and to see our love for them and our commitment to changing the world for them, even if this was not convenient for other people or for certain pharmaceutical or advocacy organizations, although I am too polite to name names. She didn't back off even if our work made us look like we were extreme angry powerful potent loving *and organized* women, which we were, and which she helped us become.

Barbara helped hundreds of us over the years to dedicate

ourselves to real solutions, instead of to nice pink feel-good gestures. She taught us to take more profound actions by getting real, by being as alive as we could possibly be.

She saved more individual lives with her wisdom, expertise, and contacts than anyone else I know. A number of women I know were diagnosed with more aggressive forms of breast cancer and were basically told that they would get a recurrence; they thwarted mainstream breast cancer doctors and modalities and instead learned about themselves, and their disease, and their health, and other women with the same cancers—and are still thriving. I loved that when someone I knew got sick, I could say, "Oh, my god, just call Barbara Brenner. Just call BCA."

Then she got sick herself, and her works, collected in this book, will show you the evolution from a woman advocating for the whole world to a woman advocating for herself in the deeply confusing world of illness. She was an extraordinary writer of clarity, brilliance, truth, humor, and heart. Now and forever, you and I can say, "Here!" and shove this book into the hands of anyone who needs Barbara. In this book, there is something true for each person who is walking through the strange Congo of breast cancer, of diagnosis, fear, limbo, treatment, recovery, and all the different ways in which we heal. This book will help thousands of people learn—and want—to be molecules, motes in a beam of light and warmth in which sick people and their compadres, survivors, and budding activists can walk, and sing, and share the sometimes tough and sometimes exhilarating truth that was, and is, the life of my sister girl Barbara.

Here is the final paragraph from the last of several stories I wrote about our friendship, her work, and her last weeks here in the visible realms. Susie and Barbara and I were taking a walk at Muir Woods, and Barbara was quietly, wildly, lovingly alive:

> Barbara pointed out a bird so tiny that Susie and I didn't see
> it at first in the fallen branches and duff of the forest floor. It
> was the only thing moving besides the humans. All of a sudden
> we saw a tiny jumpy camouflaged creature, heard the teeny
> tinkly peep. We did the obeisance of delight. A great Bay arch
> across the dirt was our last stop on the way. It was in full curvy

stretch, arched all the way over our path, reaching for sun and touching the ground on the other side. I wondered if it would snake along on top of the duff, always following the light. It is nobody's fool. Lithe and sinewy, the branch looked Asian: I guess we're all Pacific Rim on this bus. All of its leaves were gone, as if it had spent its time and life force in the arching. Barbara trundled along up to it, smiled, and made the exact arch with her hand—like, Here's the arch and I'm saluting it, standing beneath it, and now walking through.

Barbara Brenner (1951–2013) was a renowned breast cancer activist and the executive director of Breast Cancer Action. She died from ALS at the age of sixty-one.

Barbara Sjoholm is an author and translator. She cofounded and was an editor and publisher of Seal Press.

Rachel Morello-Frosch, a member of the scientific advisory board of Breast Cancer Action, is a professor in the Department of Environmental Science, Policy, and Management at the University of California, Berkeley.

Anne Lamott is the author, most recently, of *Small Victories,* which includes an essay about Barbara Brenner.

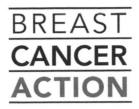

BREAST
CANCER
ACTION

Breast Cancer Action is a national education and activist organization and the watchdog for the breast cancer movement. It was founded in 1990 by a group of women living with—and dying from—breast cancer who were angry about the lack of information available about their disease. BCAction's mission is to achieve health justice for all women at risk of and living with breast cancer. Recognized for its fierce independence and unapologetic advocacy for women's health, BCAction was the first national breast cancer organization to adopt a strict corporate contributions policy in order to stay accountable to the needs of patients rather than corporate interests. For more information, go to www.bcaction.org or call (877) 278-6722.